D1595283

HANG
— THE —
BANNER

THE PROVEN GOLF FITNESS
PROGRAM USED BY THE BEST
GOLFERS IN THE WORLD

JOEY DIOVISALVI
KOLBY TULLIER
STEVE STEINBERG

ISBN: 978-0-578-32641-2 (Hardcover)
ISBN: 978-0-578-35668-6 (Paperback)
ISBN: 978-0-578-35669-3 (Electronic)

Cover and Book Design by Stephanie Fernandez

Cover photography, left to right, via Getty Images;
Sam Greenwood, Kyodo News, Sam Greenwood,
Warren Little, and Hunter Martin.

Interior photography by Cristina Martinez,
Kolby Tullier, and Mark Amuso.

Printed by Hit It Great Media, LLC, in the United States of America.

Hit It Great® Media, LLC
2885 Jupiter Park Drive #300 • Jupiter • FL • 33458
info@hititgreat.com
hititgreat.com

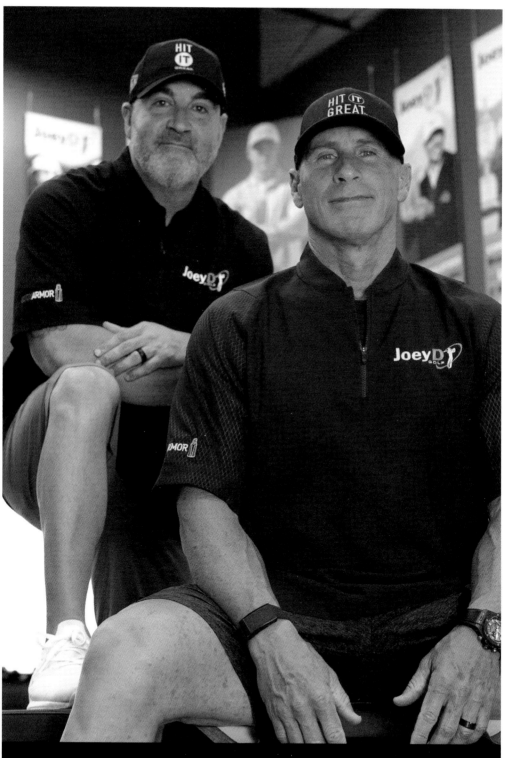

Coaches Kolby Tullier and Joey Diovisalvi

Table of Contents

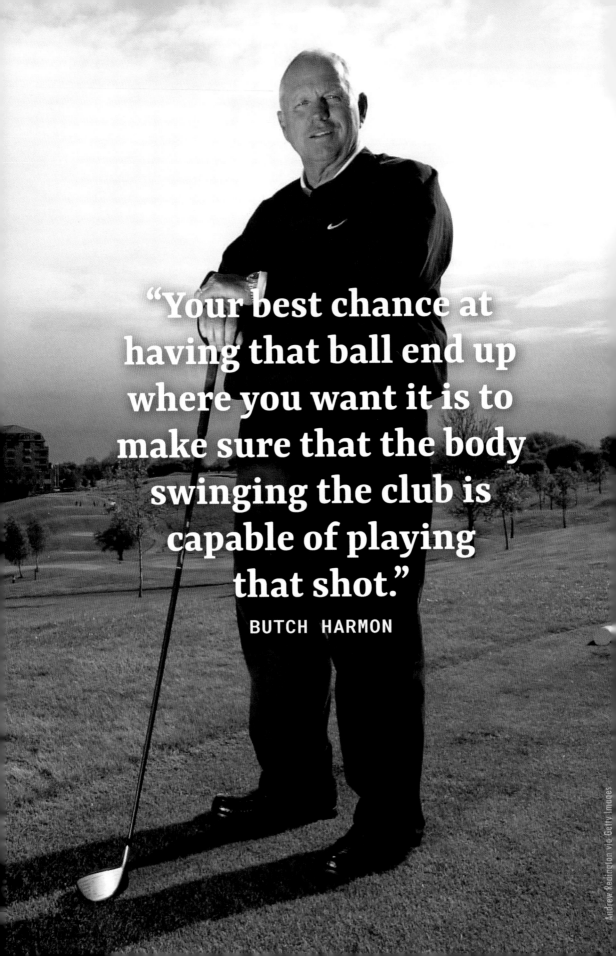

"Your best chance at having that ball end up where you want it is to make sure that the body swinging the club is capable of playing that shot."

BUTCH HARMON

Foreword

I've had the privilege of being a teaching professional for over 50 years. And I've been around golf my entire life. I watched my father share advice with Ben Hogan and I've been able to work with the likes of Tiger Woods, Greg Norman, and Dustin Johnson. One of the things that's let me stay in this game for so long is that I don't give in to fads, trends, and "magical secrets to thirty more yards off the tee." If something works, then I'm all for it. If something is new and flashy and different for the sake of being different, I stay away from it.

When I first saw Joey D working with some of his players in the PGA Tour fitness trailer, my first impression was here was something new and flashy and different for the sake of being different. Here was this intense, jacked guy with forearms that looked like rotisserie chickens putting pro golfers through workouts that didn't look like workouts that pro golfers should be doing.

The general belief had always been that strength training and weightlifting would tighten guys up. Golf isn't a strength sport; it's a sport of body control and physical nuance. It's about staying loose – not being tight. Tiger got away with a fairly strict training regimen, but Tiger is Tiger. To see these other guys doing some serious strength training, though, initially didn't make a whole lot of sense to me.

And then those guys that I saw in the trailer started to get better. They weren't going out and winning every Sunday, but they were making cuts more regularly and finishing higher up on the leaderboard. Later on, when Joey and I started to work with some of the same players, I saw firsthand how the changes he made in players' bodies made them better at being able to do the things that I wanted them to do with the club.

Players became better able to stabilize and balance and get deeper rotation where they needed it. And, suddenly, the things that weren't quite transferring over from the range to the course started transferring. Small subtle swing modifications were now resulting in major improvements. The work they were doing with Joey was making my job easier. If you're working with a swing coach or the pro at your club, they'll thank you for doing the things you'll read about in this book.

This program isn't about working out for the sake of working out; this is results-driven training with a purpose. If a player can't maintain his spine angle at the top of his backswing for a certain shot, he's not going to be able to play that shot. Ever. It's as simple as that. But if he can do things in the gym that'll allow him to maintain that spine angle, then he'll be able to play that shot. And if he puts in enough practice time on the range, that shot becomes another weapon in his arsenal. And if it's that shot that he needs to hit late on a Sunday afternoon to close out a tournament, then it's the things that he's done with Joey and Joey's people that's the difference between a trophy and a giant check and no trophy and, well, a still-pretty-big check.

But this isn't just for the players you see on TV. This is for anyone who wants to get better at the sport of golf. The ball doesn't move on its own and the club doesn't move on its own. It's the player who swings the club and it's that split second at impact that determines where the club is going to send the ball. Your best chance at having that ball end up where you want it is to make sure that the body swinging the club is capable of playing that shot. And it's the things in this book that'll allow that to happen.

– **Butch Harmon**

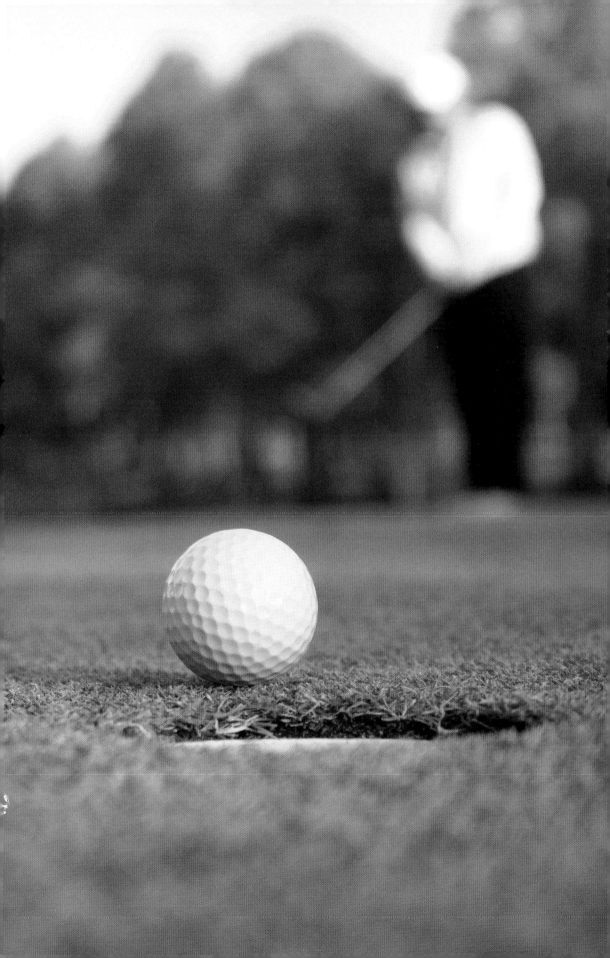

"Reverse every natural instinct and do the opposite of what you are inclined to do, and you will probably come very close to having a perfect golf swing."

BEN HOGAN

Introduction

Man has been writing about how to better his golf game – and complaining about his inability to do so – for almost as long as man has been playing golf. And, amazingly, the things we were writing about and were frustrated with almost a century and a half ago are the same things that we're still writing about and still frustrated with – distance, accuracy, and trying to swing the club like the best players in the game.

Way back in 1887, Sir Walter G. Simpson wrote about the problems facing the typical player in his book, *The Art of Golf*: "They see the professional's club swishing around his back, and they determine, at all costs, to get theirs as far around. By a variety of schemes they accomplish this, and become the proud possessors of a concatenation of contortions, in which no one but themselves recognizes to a full swing."

Fast-forward over a century and we still see all the compensations players come up with to try to make their swings more effective and more powerful. They open their stance. They close their stance. They lean. They sway. And they do something you couldn't even do in 1887 – they go out and drop $700 on a new driver.

When you read what was written over a hundred years ago, it's mind-boggling that we're even still playing golf today – or that the sport wasn't simply outlawed! In 1914, Henry Leach compared golf to a fistfight in his book, *The Happy Golfer*: "The difference between golf and fisticuffs is that in the one the pain is of the mind and in the other it is of the body."

In a way it's kind of comforting to know that if your great-grandfather was a golfer, he probably wanted to snap a club over his knee just as often as you want to. Heck, for a lot of players, what golf instructor Alex J. Morrison wrote in *A New Way to Better Golf* back in 1932 is still the most accurate line ever written about the sport: "It is only at the nineteenth hole that the average golfer enjoys any relaxation."

While a lot has changed in the past 150 years, a few things haven't. The golf swing remains one of the most complicated movements in all of sports. And golfers are still looking for direction on the road to success and still incredibly frustrated at how difficult the game can be.

We know this because we've spent a combined 50 years helping golfers play better golf. We know that the golf club doesn't swing itself and that if your goal is to swing the club better, the fastest and most effective way to do that is to optimize the body that swings that club. And by "optimizing," we're being very specific. We're not optimizing the body for running triathlons. We're not optimizing the body for playing tennis. We're optimizing the body for swinging a golf club.

A few years ago, Coach Joey Diovisalvi decided to put his own mark on the literary world. His best-selling book on golf biomechanics, *Fix Your Body, Fix Your Swing*, forever changed the perception of golf fitness. It began a revolution in the way that golfers – from PGA and LPGA pros to weekend players – looked at and understood the importance of strength and movement.

Hang the Banner adds Kolby "K-Wayne" Tullier into the mix. Kolby has been helping top athletes reach their potential for over 20 years and has spent the last 10 years working with PGA and LPGA Tour pros like Justin Thomas, Lexi Thompson, Michelle Wie, Lucas Glover, and Harold Varner, III.

If you want to think of *Fix Your Body, Fix Your Swing* as a troubleshooting guide for the golfer's body, then *Hang the Banner* is the instruction manual on how to build that body from scratch.

You're only going to swing the club as well as your body will allow you to swing the club, so we've broken the body down joint-by-joint to help you see exactly where your body isn't letting you swing the club correctly. Once you eliminate the weak links in the way your body moves, you've eliminated the things that are preventing you from swinging the club the way you want to.

For proof that our system works, you only have to step foot in the Joey D Golf Sports Training Center in Jupiter, Florida. At any given time, you might see a present or former world number one working out side by side with a top LPGA player, a rising high school star, or someone who just picked up a club for the first time last week.

As of this writing, the top three American golfers – Brooks Koepka, Justin Thomas, and Dustin Johnson – all train at the facility. At one point, they've all been number one in the world. Let that sink in for a minute. The top three male golfers in the country – not to mention the dozens of other world-ranked PGA and LPGA Tour players – all work out under the same roof using the same training protocols and philosophies. That just doesn't happen in other sports. Roger Federer and Rafael Nadal don't train together when they get ready for Wimbledon or the US Open. And Marvin Hagler and Thomas Hearns didn't share the same gym as they prepared for their epic battle.

We like to joke that there must be something in the water in Jupiter that's taking golfers to the next level. Honestly, though, we wish it were that easy; we would have opened up a bottling plant and started shipping out six-packs years ago. But the answer isn't in the water; it's in this book.

With over a half-century of combined strength, conditioning, and biomechanics experience, we know what it takes to get a beginning player to feel comfortable with their swing. We know what it takes to help a very good player over that last hurdle so that they can win their first PGA or LPGA Tour event. And we know what it takes to move a top-10 player into the number one spot in the world.

You now have everything you need to transform your body into one that's optimized for the golf course. This is no generic workout served up alongside a healthy dose of golf jargon. This is the same workout program that the top players in the world rely on to get to – and stay at – the top of their game. This is how we build champions.

Be prepared to experience profound changes in the way you play the game of golf.

Let's get to work.

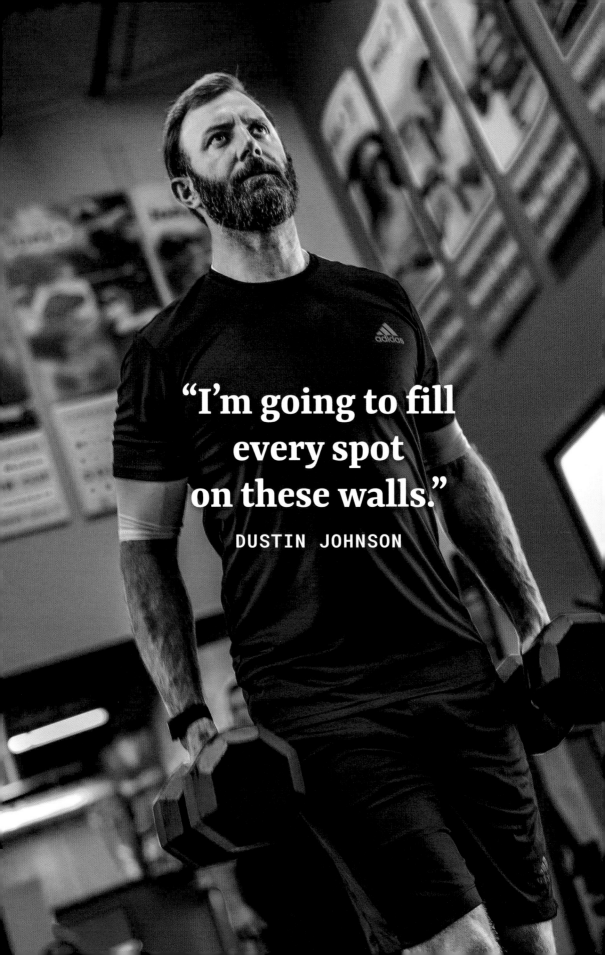

"I'm going to fill
every spot
on these walls."

DUSTIN JOHNSON

CHAPTER ONE

Hang the Banner

Interstate 95 is over 1,900 miles long and runs from the Canadian border in Maine down to Miami, Florida. The road has over 650 exits that give you access to everything from lobsters in New England and crab cakes in Maryland to fireworks in South Carolina and real-life rocket ships in Cape Canaveral.

Exit 78 in St. George, South Carolina, is where you want to jump off if you're heading to Augusta for The Masters and either Exit 329 or the Florida 202 exit in Jacksonville, Florida, if you're heading to THE PLAYERS Championship. But if you're among the top golfers in the world – or just want to train like them – you're looking for Exit 87A in Jupiter, Florida.

The exit throws you off onto Indiantown Road. Head east on Indiantown for about a mile, passing one of the world's best Starbucks on your right. Turn onto Central Boulevard and then take a right on Jupiter Park Drive and after about a half mile, pull into a small industrial office park.

Welcome to the Joey D Golf Sports Training Center.

Walk through the reception area and onto the main floor and immediately your eyes are drawn upward. Hanging high up on the 24-foot walls and ringing the room are the banners. The two-foot wide, six-foot long banners each represent a PGA, LPGA, or Korn Ferry Tour victory by one of the many golfers who work out here. Past the main floor is the larger workout area, and the walls there are also ringed with banners. As of this writing, we've hung more than 50 banners on the walls.

Nothing short of a W earns a banner. (Actually, there is one other way to earn a banner: become number one in the world. Currently, there are four of those extra-large banners hanging.)

> *"It hits me more sometimes in that gym than in real life when I see my banners up there and I get chills and I'm, like, 'Wow. That's pretty awesome.' And just to be up there with other athletes – some of the best golfers in the world – it's an honor."*
> **– Lexi Thompson**

When you walk into the TD Garden in Boston, you see the Celtics' 17 NBA Championship banners hanging from the rafters. When visiting teams see those banners, they realize that they're not only going up against the latest version of the Celtics, they're also going up against the ghosts and legacy and magnitude of those 17 past championships. We wanted to create that same aura of success and history.

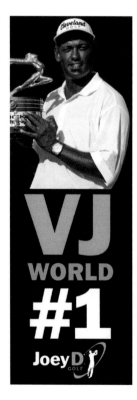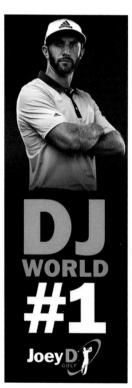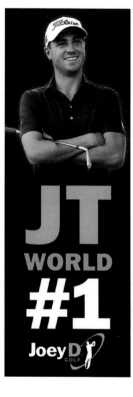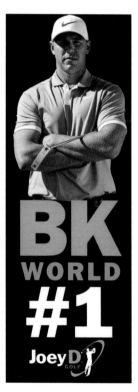

We want anyone working out here – whether they've already won a bunch of majors or they're just trying to make their high school team – to know they're in a place where champions are built. We wanted to give them visual proof that if they trust the process and put in the work, there's no goal that isn't attainable.

Unlike other sports, golf has no home games and no home stadiums or arenas. (And a lot of the most prestigious events don't even happen at the same venue year-to-year.) Players teeing it up for the PGA Championship may know in the back of their minds that Brooks Koepka has won the major twice in the past three years, but there aren't two massive and intimidating banners hanging above their heads reminding them of that fact. We wanted to be able to honor those victories and give the players that work out here a sense that this is their home. This is their clubhouse. Once they earn a banner, it's not coming down and no one can take that victory away from them.

Out on tour, players aren't just competing for a trophy and a check; they're competing for the ownership of some very coveted wall space and the bragging rights that come with it. Someone will win an event and they'll be up on the green holding a crystal trophy and a check for one-point-something million and then they'll catch sight of one of us and they'll be like, "Hey! Hang the banner!"

> *"I think the banners are really important and I think it's such a cool thing to do. It's definitely motivation. It was awesome to see my first banner up there especially since I was up there with my friends Marina and Jessica."*
> – **Michelle Wie**

They're also a great motivational tool. A player who is hungry for a win might "conveniently" get positioned so that all he can see is Dustin Johnson's banners while he works out. And that's all he'll be able to look at for the entire hour. They're also about respect. People may know that DJ has won 24 times on the PGA Tour, but when you see all those banners and realize that each one represents not only the four-day grind that it took to win the event, but the countless hours of work that went in just to be able to compete at that level, it can be daunting. We wanted to create that atmosphere of respect that you have in other sports. We want the guy coming in who just got his Tour card to feel like the NBA or NFL rookie who reports to the first day of training camp and discovers his locker is right next to a future Hall of Famer.

"You go in and there are all these banners of world number ones, FedEx champions, and major champions and it makes you feel like you're a part of something that's bigger than you. I see DJ or Justin Thomas or Joaquin (Niemann) every time I'm there. So, you're not just seeing their banners, you're seeing their faces. And they're working hard, and it makes you realize how much harder you have to work to be where they are."
– **Talor Gooch**

The facility opened in 2012 as a 2,000-square-foot box with weights, resistance bands, and a bunch of other toys. There was one goal: to help golfers optimize their bodies for the sport of golf. If that wasn't your goal, there was no reason to be there. It was a risky venture in the already risky-venture-filled fitness industry. Sort of like opening up a restaurant and only serving one dish. Generally, that's not a smart business model. Or, if it is, it's a temporary one. Folks get their fill of that one dish – the best noodle soup ever, the best thin-crust pizza ever, whatever – and then move on to the next culinary fad.

Unlike man's limited appetite for designer grilled cheese sandwiches, though, the demand for golf-specific training and conditioning never waned. Two thousand square feet became 4,000 square feet, which became 8,000 square feet. Currently, Joey D Golf weighs in at a lofty 10,000 square feet and all eyes are on the various walls that we'll need to knock down for further expansion.

And while an increase in business and demand is the primary reason for the growth of the facility, the number of Tour wins by the athletes working out in the facility is another one; we just need more wall space for banners.

"There are so many banners up and DJ and Justin are taking over the front room and it's so annoying. It makes everyone else want to put their little dent in the room, so it's fun. When somebody wins, you just wait for that banner to go up. It's a pride thing. In a sense, it's a very individual sport, but Kolby calls us all his 'stable,' so it's a little bit of a family, as well."
– **Jessica Korda**

The training center's exponential growth from such a humble beginning is made even more impressive when you consider the fact that in 2012, most people didn't even consider golfers to be athletes. A golfer working with weights was considered a novelty. The media used to question what we did: why would a golfer need to work with a strength, conditioning, and biomechanics coach? To them, it was legitimate journalism. To us, it was a slap in the face – as if everything we were doing in the gym or out on the road with players was a façade and an enormous waste of time. The argument was that the golf swing was more of a technique than an athletic movement. Wisely, we – mostly – held our tongues in check and stated our side of the argument delicately and with as much poise as possible.

Fortunately, we rarely have to practice such incredible self-control anymore. Few people question the idea of the golfer as an athlete anymore. It doesn't matter if you're talking about the PGA Tour, the LPGA Tour, or the Champions Tour, there's no denying that the players who are winning these days are bigger, stronger, and more fit than the players who were winning several years ago. We like to think that, in some small way, we played a part in this, but the reality is that the sport itself is responsible for it. As players get better, the competition has to get better if it wants to stay in the game. And the bar is constantly being raised.

"I'm going to fill every spot on these walls." – **Dustin Johnson**

In an indirect way, every lunge that Brooks Koepka does makes Lexi Thompson a better player, and every rotational drill that Jessica Korda does makes Justin Thomas a better player. Golf used to have the reputation of being a "gentlemen's game," but at the highest level of the sport, it's now athletes playing golf; it's not gentlemen playing golf. The competition is fierce and everyone can hit the ball far. Courses wouldn't be forced to play bigger and longer every year if this was all just a bunch of nonathletes showing off their techniques. And that applies to the LPGA Tour, Korn Ferry Tour, D1 college golf, and the American Junior Golf Association (AJGA), as well.

The fact is that any athletic movement is essentially a technique. Hitting a baseball, throwing a punch, kicking a football are all techniques. Once you've gotten pretty good at that technique, you improve its effectiveness by being able to do it harder, faster, and with more control. Hitting a golf ball is no different. In less than two seconds, Dustin Johnson goes from an essentially frozen, statue-like address to a post-shot, coiled follow-through. And in that split second of movement, he's sent a 1.68-inch diameter ball over 300 yards away and landed it within a few yards of his target on a narrow fairway. How is that any different from a Nolan Ryan, Pedro Martinez, or Aroldis Chapman rearing back and firing a 103-mph fastball that paints the inside corner?

And it's no different with your game and your swing. You're only going to be able to swing the club as effectively as your body will allow you to. It's as simple as that. The key to improving your game is to make your body as efficient as possible at swinging the club properly. To do that requires a plan and a blueprint that takes into account both overall human movement patterns and golf-specific movement patterns. This is that plan. This is that blueprint.

You can know anatomy, but if you don't know how to apply that knowledge, nothing is going to improve. Biomechanics is an applied science. And no one has a better track record of applying the laws of biomechanics to the game of golf than we do. No one. Everything that you're about to do is exactly what the best golfers in the world do to stay at the top of their game. These are not random workouts and this is not guesswork. This is a results-driven, scientific approach to optimizing your body to perform one of the most complex movements in all of sports.

You see the phrase "Tour-proven" thrown around all the time. Some pair of sunglasses or golf glove is touted as Tour-proven just because a player or two or ten might use those glasses or that glove on the PGA or LPGA Tour. Wonderful. You may end up looking a fraction more like a pro player, but will those glasses or that glove really have an impact on the way you play? Will your game improve drastically or dramatically because you're wearing a certain pair of sunglasses or a certain glove? Probably not.

We don't take the phrase "Tour-proven" lightly.

Here's what Tour-proven means to us:

Tour-proven is that between February 19, 2017 and February 9, 2020 – almost three full calendar years – either Dustin Johnson, Brooks Koepka, or Justin Thomas held the World Number One ranking for 142 out of 155 weeks. For almost three straight years, the best golfer in the world worked out in Jupiter using the same golf-optimizing fitness program that you're about to embark on. Three. Straight. Years.

Tour-proven is that DJ, Justin, and Brooks were named PGA Tour Player of the Year for 2016, 2017, and 2018, respectively and that DJ and Justin split Player of the Year honors in 2020 – DJ winning the award from the PGA Tour and JT winning it from the PGA of America.

Tour-proven is that Lexi Thompson was named LPGA Player of the Year for 2017.

Tour-proven is three straight U.S. Open titles and back-to-back PGA Championships.

Tour-proven is that Justin Thomas won the FedEx Cup in 2017, while in that same year, Lexi Thompson won the CME Group Tour Championship, the LPGA's equivalent.

Tour-proven is that Dustin Johnson won the FedEx Cup in 2020.

Tour-proven is that Dustin Johnson wasn't content to simply win the FedEx Cup in 2020. Two months later, he won the COVID-delayed Masters with a course record 268.

Tour-proven is Tour wins by Jessica Korda, Michelle Wie, Marina Alex, Scott Piercy, Joaquin Niemann, Richy Werenski, and Austin Ernst. And more top-five and top-ten finishes than we can count by these players and by others you'll hear from throughout the book.

Tour-proven is Lucas Glover, who won the U.S. Open at Bethpage Black in 2009, and at age 40 had one of his best seasons ever.

Tour-proven is what happened the first week in August 2020 – a rare week when there was both a World Golf Championships event and a PGA Tour event. Justin Thomas and Brooks Koepka finished first and second at the WGC FedEx-St. Jude International and Richy Werenski won the title at the Barracuda Championship.

Heck, Tour-proven is the fact that we keep having to edit and update the stats in this book while we're writing it, because players keep winning.

And while we're as proud as can be of all the pros that work out with us, we're just as proud – or maybe more so – of all the juniors, seniors, and recreational golfers that have improved their game at our facility. They see the success that literally surrounds them while they work out. They know that to succeed, they – just like the best players in the world – have to trust the process. Trust, train, and win. That's all we ask. And there's no reason why you can't take the proven blueprint for success you're holding in your hands and elevate your game to the next level, shoot lower scores, and have a lot more fun out on the course. We not only see the results of this training every day at the Joey D Golf Sports Training Center, but we also see it late in the afternoon on just about every Sunday of the golf season.

And we've even hung some banners as proof.

> *"Right now, there are two chains holding the spot for whoever gets the next banner. The bolts are there and everything. And I'm like 'Man, I want that to be my spot.'"* – **Jaye Marie Green**

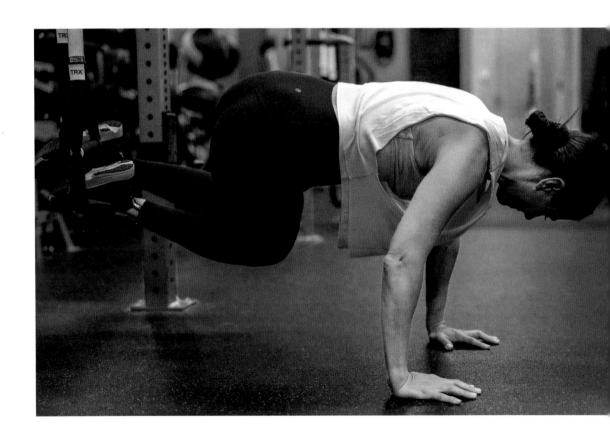

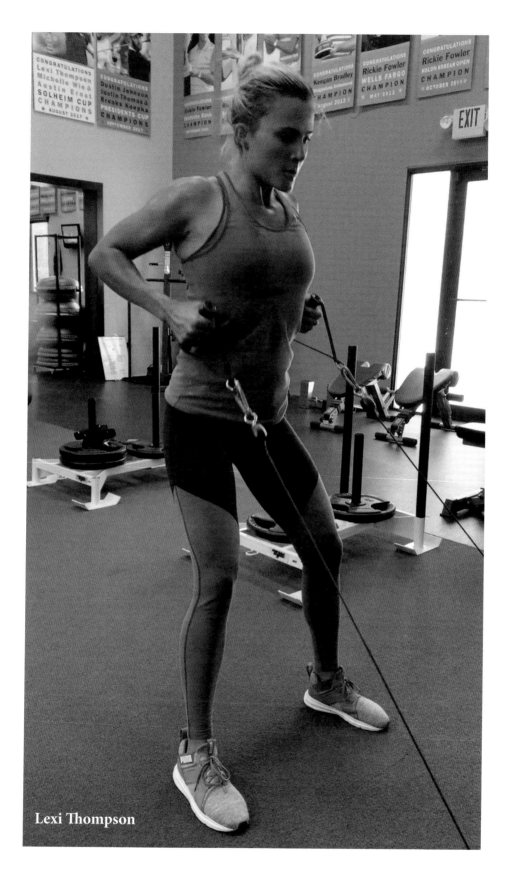

Lexi Thompson

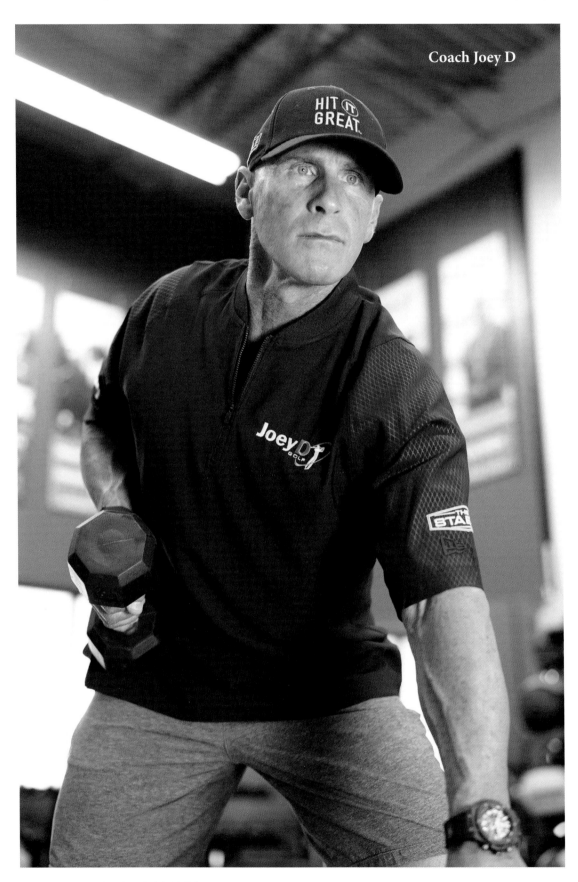

Coach Joey D

CHAPTER TWO

The Coaches

"COACH JOEY D" DIOVISALVI

My passion for fitness and movement was originally about trying to become the best athlete I could possibly be. But sometimes life has other ideas for you.

When I was about 13, I got my first set of weights – a 110-pound set of sand-filled weights that I'm sure plenty of you might have also thrown around as a kid. I loved challenging my body. I loved seeing what I could – and couldn't – do. I loved being able to do something that I wasn't able to do a week or two weeks earlier. Genetically, I was pretty lucky. My body responded really well to strength training. By the time I was 15, I had outgrown the sand-filled weights and had graduated to Olympic plates. I was 5' 5" and 180 pounds and was convinced I could go rep for rep with just about anyone else at the gym.

I brought that same competitive fire into whatever sports I played. And I played most of them growing up. I wrestled, I did martial arts, I ran track, I played soccer and baseball. Mainly, though, I played football. I'm not sure what it was about the game – the intensity, the strategy, the contact – that hooked me, but in my mid-teens, there were only two seasons for me: football season and getting-ready-for-football season.

I grew up in Manalapan, New Jersey. If you lived in the area at the time, you would have seen this strange kid running up and down hills all day and into the night in July and August. That would have been me getting ready for the football season. Despite the fact that I knew that every other kid was home watching TV or doing something else, I was convinced that I had to push myself and that I had to work harder. The end result wasn't hard to predict. I was already physically much stronger than everyone else my age and when you add to that this insane drive that I had inside me, the result was that I was just a beast in every game. My coach had to sit me at half-time because the other team couldn't stop me. Eventually, parents and coaches from other teams said they wanted to see my birth certificate, because they couldn't believe that a 13- or 14-year-old kid was doing what I was doing.

By the time I was 18, I was almost 200 pounds and I had done it all without shortcuts. Steroids were all over the place at the time, but they never made sense to me. Not only were they cheating, but they were incredibly dangerous. I've always been very aware of what I put into my body. I've never drank and I've never smoked. And if I have one vice, it's Starbucks – more specifically, it's an iced grande Americano with extra water and extra ice in a venti cup. (Try it sometime.)

Through hard work, dedication, and sacrifice, I built my body into the perfect football-playing machine and I was convinced that one day I'd be playing in the NFL.

To quote Mike Tyson: "Everyone has a plan until they get punched in the mouth."

Shortly before my 19th birthday, I discovered a lump on my right testicle. A close family friend, who was a doctor, examined me and gave me the number of an oncologist and told me to call him as soon as I could. It was the beginning of a medical nightmare that ripped apart my world. The first surgery I had was a biopsy. It was a painful procedure that was horrendous on so many levels. The only positive was that, in my mind, it was done, it was over, and I was convinced that I'd have my life back and be able to get back into the gym and back onto the football field.

A few days later, the doctor called and said he needed to see me. The biopsy results weren't good. The tumor they removed was malignant and the cancer had spread to my lymph nodes. He said it had advanced past the point where he could help and he gave me the names of some doctors that he thought would be willing to try some last-ditch and experimental procedures on me. My mind was a blur. And all I really remember after that was him telling me that surgery was no guarantee of success, but if I didn't have surgery, he could guarantee that I'd be dead within a year.

Two weeks later, I was back in the operating room for back-to-back procedures that would take the better parts of two days and leave me unconscious for another two days. I can't imagine it being physically possible to feel any worse than I did when I finally woke up. The doctor told me I was a very lucky man, but I wasn't feeling particularly lucky at that moment. And then chemotherapy started. At the time, it wasn't an outpatient procedure. It was a hellish seven straight days of in-hospital treatment every three weeks for six months. I was sick, weak, and nauseous around-the-clock the entire time. I dropped from a massive 200 pounds to a frail 165 pounds. But, eventually, I was declared cancer-free.

I slowly began the process of rebuilding my body, my strength, and my life. It was a lot of work and pain and a lot of frustration and setbacks. I had never been someone who lacked confidence in my abilities or who lacked motivation, but there were so many times when it would have been so easy just to give up. But if you believe in the process, you continue to grind. Ultimately, it was a profoundly life-affirming experience. The same movements and exercises that used to be about getting better on the football field were now about being able to move like a regular person and regain a normal life.

Everything took on a new context. My time in the gym, which had always been so important to me, now took on an almost religious significance. Thanks to the power of movement and the power of exercise, I was able to claw my way back from the

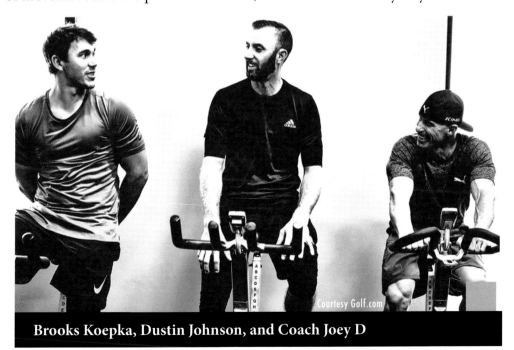

Brooks Koepka, Dustin Johnson, and Coach Joey D

almost-dead. But whatever dreams I had for a career in sports were probably over. I don't want to get too cocky or profound and say it was a calling, but I knew that if I could rebuild a body and life ravaged by cancer and chemotherapy, I could probably help just about anyone.

I moved to South Florida and began working as a trainer. My intensity, work ethic, motivational skills, and attention to detail gelled with a lot of the pro athletes who either lived in the area or spent their off-seasons there. As a student of the human body, I was like a kid in a candy store. I was working with 6' 10" basketball players, pitchers who could throw a baseball in the high 90s, and runners who could steal bases with blinding speed. On a daily basis, I was studying and analyzing elite athletic performance. And then coming up with ways to make that performance even more impressive.

My reputation began to spread. In the late 90s, I got a call from the late, great Clarence Clemons – the legendary sax player from Bruce Springsteen's E Street Band. He had just had surgery and wanted some help with his recovery. I ended up going on tour with the band and working with everyone from Clarence and guitarists Nils Lofgren and Steven Van Zandt to Bruce and his wife, Patti.

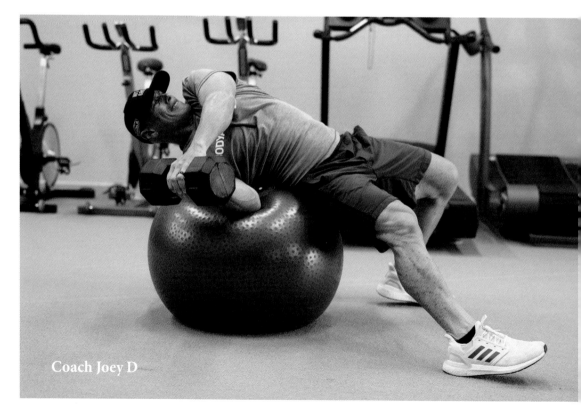

Coach Joey D

And, yeah, there aren't too many things cooler than being a kid from Jersey and being on tour with Springsteen. It was unlike anything I'd ever experienced up to that point. But when the tour ended, I found myself entering another world that was just as foreign and just as intriguing: the world of professional golf. I had gotten a call from my friend, Eric Hillcoff, saying that golfer Jesper Parnevik was looking to work with someone who could strengthen his body for the game. Little did I know where this would lead me!

While other sports had developed complex sport-specific training philosophies and protocols to improve performance, the sport of golf in the year 2001 seemed stuck in the past. Sure, Gary Player was always talking about the virtues of fitness for golfers and there was a young Tiger Woods, who clearly looked like he knew his way around the gym, but there wasn't nearly the same focus on strength, conditioning, and biomechanics that there was in most every other sport. For the most part, the fitness trailer on the PGA Tour was the place where players stretched out and got massages.

Work with Jesper Parnevik and others led to me meeting and training Vijay Singh and eventually moving up to Ponte Vedra to work with him exclusively. Working with Vijay on a day-to-day basis was eye-opening. During our time together, I must have watched him hit a half-million golf balls. I was able to break down the movement patterns of the golf swing and come up with exercises and drills designed to optimize the body's ability to perform those movement patterns. And since Vijay had one of the greatest work ethics of anyone I've ever been around, his body quickly adapted to the changes we were demanding of it and his game got better.

In 2004, Vijay's win at the Deutsche Bank Championship moved him past Tiger Woods and into the number one spot in the world. It was an amazing feeling to be part of such a successful team. CBS Sports did a TV special about the training we had been doing to get his body in optimal condition to play. They showed us running on the beach playing medicine ball catch and some other things that would be considered pretty normal by today's standards. Back then, though, it was considered off-the-wall and I was portrayed as some mad scientist. In a way it was cool to be recognized for what we were accomplishing, but, at the same time, it was a drag to be considered somewhat of a sideshow.

By 2010, I needed a break from the road. I was traveling 25-plus weeks out of the year while working with seven or eight different pros on tour. My usually through-the-roof intensity level was starting to lag. I was tired of waking up at 4:30 in the morning and not knowing what city I was in. I was tired of never seeing the house I owned in Jacksonville. I was tired of just being tired. My book, *Fix Your Body, Fix Your Swing*, had just been released. And I had successfully transitioned from being the nut running on the beach with Vijay Singh to being the guy behind "the revolutionary biomechanics program used by tour pros." I moved back down to South Florida and opened up the Joey D Golf Sports Training Center in Jupiter.

It was a game-changer. I was no longer limited by the space and equipment in the Tour trailer or in the hotel gyms we were forced to use when we were on the road. I could finally build a gym that looked and felt exactly how I wanted. And, as usual, my goal was simple and humble: I wanted to have the best golf-specific training facility in the world.

The last piece of the puzzle fell into place a few years later in Dallas, Texas. I was introduced to Kolby Tullier, who was working with Justin Thomas and a few other players. We sat down and talked and he told me that between us – with our knowledge, experience, and vision – we could change the world. We could change the way golfers trained, and we could change the way the world looked at golfers and their athleticism. And Kolby was more than just talk. He didn't waver and he didn't procrastinate. He was so convinced that we could flip the golf world upside-down that he uprooted his family from Louisiana and moved to Jupiter. And together – and with the help of some great coaches and club fitters – we've made the Joey D Golf Sports Training Center the best golf-specific training facility in the world.

Looking back, there were so many times when the train could have jumped the track and I wouldn't be where I am right now. I'm older and wiser now, but my belief in the power of movement and the power of exercise has never waned. I still work out seven days a week, and I still love challenging my body. And I'm fortunate to be able to make a living getting others to challenge theirs. I know what the human body is capable of. And I get no greater joy than helping someone find that extra gear they didn't know they had and helping them tap into the hidden strengths – both physical and mental – that will make them a better person and a better player.

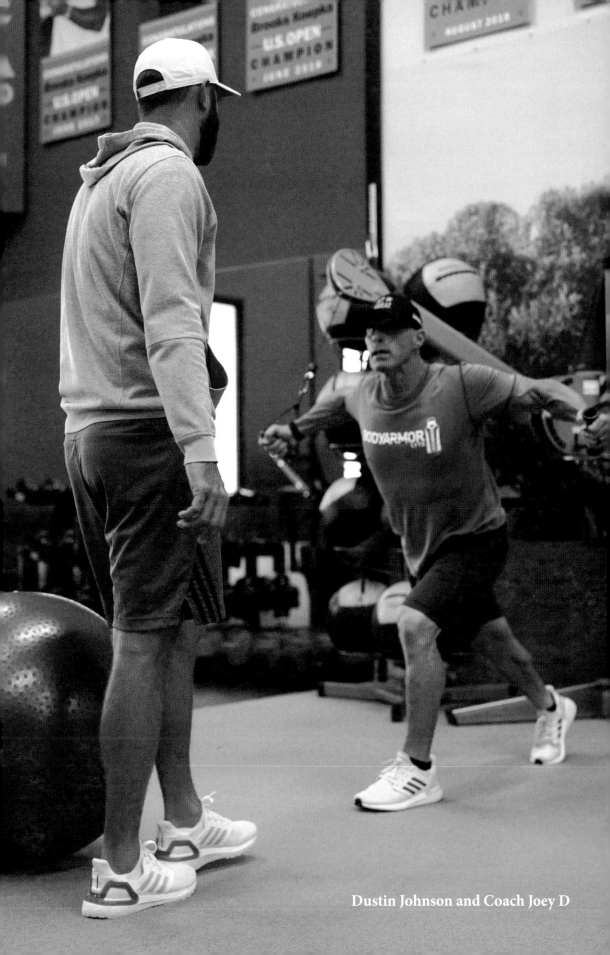

Dustin Johnson and Coach Joey D

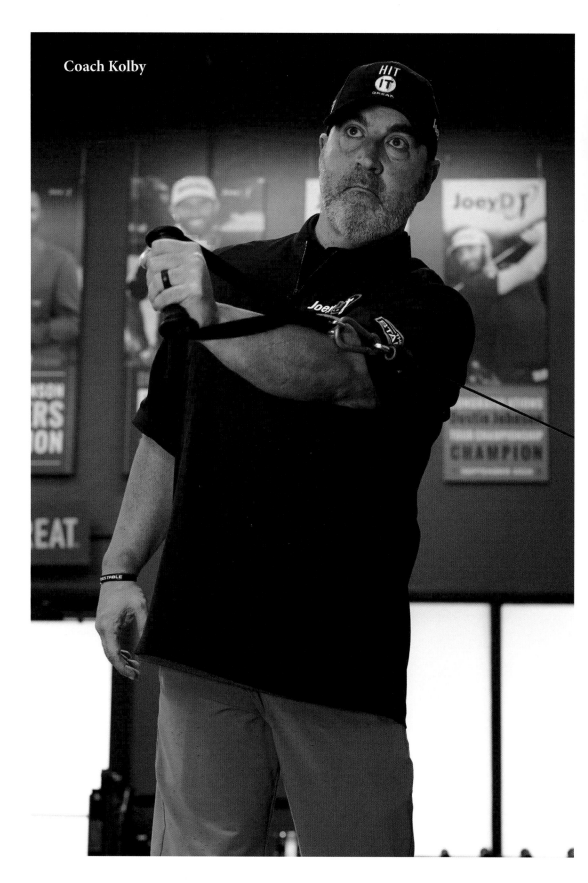

Coach Kolby

KOLBY "COACH K-WAYNE" TULLIER

I didn't take the typical road to becoming a fitness professional. My obsession with human movement and performance started at a very early age. And, originally, it was more about necessity than anything else.

I was born crippled. I was born with two club feet in 1975. The doctors saw it immediately when I was born and just whisked me out of the operating room. My mother never even got a chance to see me. She was expecting everything to be like the scene in a movie where she's sitting up in her hospital bed and they bring in a beautiful baby all clean and wrapped up and there's a smiling nurse saying, "Congratulations! It's a boy!" But that never happened. Instead, a doctor eventually came in and told my parents that I'd probably never walk.

Now that I have a little girl of my own, I can't imagine what that must have been like for them.

To the doctors' credit, while my mother was waiting to see her brand-new baby, they were already busy trying to figure out what to do with an infant whose feet were both so horribly curved in and curled up that they looked like a lowercase B and a lowercase D. They had begun searching into specialists who they thought would be able to help, but in the meantime, they just put my feet in casts – which they had to change every week for nine months straight. It was just the beginning of an entire childhood spent in casts.

Specialists came in from all over the nation to look at this deformed little baby from outside of Baton Rouge, but it was a doctor from the Crippled Children's Hospital in New Orleans who really thought he could help. His ideas were sort of on the cutting edge and he had an experimental surgery that he wanted to try. I had my first surgery as an infant in 1977. It was the first of four surgeries that I had all the way through high school.

And even though it wasn't all that long ago, looking back, the procedures seem very severe. They'd cut across the tops of my feet and try to turn and straighten my feet a little bit more. Then they would put me in casts all the way up to my waist so that I wouldn't be able to move and mess up what they'd done reconstructively. One time, they took a piece of bone out of my hip, cut it in half, and inserted it into my feet to help create an ankle. After another surgery, I was able to walk, but my heels weren't touching the ground, so they went back in, broke both of my feet and stuck pins through my heels.

And after every surgery, I had to relearn how to walk.

I remember when I was little, my grandmother did a lot of the taking care of me. My mother had to go to work because of all the added expenses my surgeries and recovery were costing. I would look outside and see the other kids, like my brother and sister, playing and I'd start to get really sad. To say I was crying would probably be an understatement. And she would straighten me up quickly. "Stop that crying," she'd say. And then she'd tell me, "God put you on this Earth to teach people how to be strong." I remember it like it was yesterday. At the time, it probably didn't make much sense to me. How was I going to teach people to be strong when I couldn't even go outside to play with the other kids? Instead, she would drag me around the house on a blanket because I couldn't walk.

Relearning how to walk after each surgery was exhausting and frustrating, but, ultimately, it was an incredible lesson in perseverance. Because of the casts and being

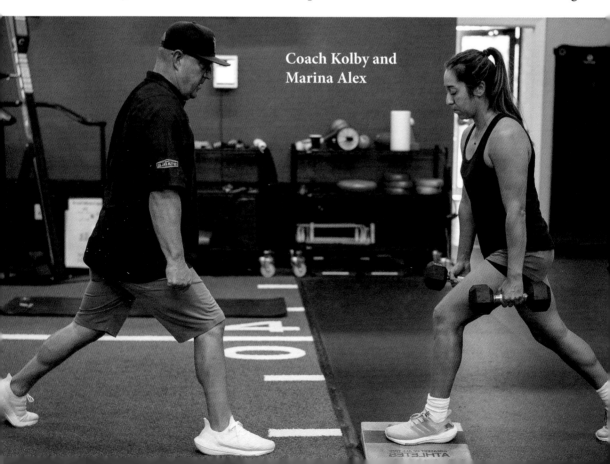

Coach Kolby and Marina Alex

unable to move a lot, all the muscles in my legs and feet had atrophied. So, when I wasn't in casts, I'd have on these Forrest Gump-looking leg braces or bar braces or whatever crazy gadgets the doctors thought would help. At one point, I looked like a stormtrooper from *Star Wars* because the braces were white and they would come up out of my shoes and all the way up my leg. It seems that half my life until I was about 15 was spent in leg braces holding on to poles trying to walk a straight line.

There were so many doctor's appointments. And this wasn't like the average person going to see their doctor and getting a "Hey, how are you doing?" I would go for checkups and there'd be all these doctors from all over the world looking at my feet and trying to learn how to fix people like me. I was the lab rat. I'm actually in a medical book. The surgeries they do for club feet now are based on the procedures that I had over 30 years ago.

Eventually, I was walking and moving more normally. I was able to start playing some sports. I probably pushed myself too hard at times – at night I'd crawl to the bathroom, bathe, and then crawl to my bedroom – but I was trying to make up for all those years I couldn't do much.

All of this molded me into who I am now. I knew from a young age that I had to outwork everybody else because I was so different from everybody else. Life deals you a hand and you can either whine about it or you can do something about it. My parents and my family never let me feel sorry for myself. My grandmother passed away when I was five or six, but she's always been a part of me and still is to this day. And my parents were very hard-working people and everything they did sent out a message about the importance of determination and trying to better oneself.

When it was time to go to college, I got offered a full academic scholarship from Southeastern Louisiana University. It may not have been exactly where I wanted to go, but free tuition meant that it wouldn't be costing my parents any money. My original major was pre-optometry. I thought my parents would like telling people that their son was a doctor. At the same time, though, I was fascinated with physical therapy. I'd already spent half my life with physical therapists and the other half at home experimenting with my own ideas about how to get my body to feel and move better.

I got jobs at a couple of local gyms. Every morning, I'd get up and go to work at one gym and then go to school and then go to work at the other gym. It was crazy hours and a crazy lifestyle, but it's essentially the same morning to night workday that I keep today. I remember when I decided to change my major to Exercise Physiology. To my parents, I went from being a doctor to being a gym teacher. But I knew that I would be able to help people and that's what was driving me.

I got a job at a cardiac rehab facility and then later at one of the top physical therapy businesses in the state. I was able to experience amazing things. I could watch surgeries. I got to see how the shoulder really worked and how the knee really worked. I wasn't just reading about these things in a book. I was seeing them in person with my own eyes.

After I graduated with a degree in Exercise Physiology, I told my father I wanted to open a training business. My dad had worked 20-plus years on the state police force and was on the verge of retiring, but because his son had this dream of opening a training studio and changing the world, he mortgaged everything he and my mother had built together and helped me open my business. He could have retired and been living on Easy Street, but all of a sudden he's half-a-million dollars in debt.

I remember my first day of work. It was 4:30 am and he was already up. I'm in the living room putting on my shoes and he looks at me and says, "You wanted it. So go get your ass up and go get it." For three straight years, I left the house at 4:30 every morning and got home at 10:30 every night. And after three years, we'd paid off all the loans. My parents still live in that house. We have family gatherings there, and my mom will cook up a storm. She can feed the whole southern half of the state of Louisiana out of her kitchen.

I ran my business, Body Mechanics, for the next 15 years and watched it grow. Eventually, I was bought out and stayed for a year as performance director. At the time, I had started working with a few golfers like John Peterson, Andrew Loupe, and Smylie Kaufman. When they were on the road, they asked if I could join them on the Tour. That opened up a whole new world for me.

On the road, I met Joey and we just clicked. I had read his book and knew who he was. I've always been of the mindset that if you want to be successful, you find the most successful person and you learn from them. Eventually, he offered me a position at his facility in Jupiter, Florida. I thought about life in Louisiana. We were doing well. I had a good job. My wife had a good job. We had a child who was happy and in school. And one day I walked in and said, "We're moving. I'm leaving first. I'm gonna see y'all in about three months."

Since then, I've had the opportunity to work with some of the best golfers in the world. In addition, my roster of athletes from other pro sports continues to grow and includes everyone from pitchers you see throwing heat in the MLB postseason to wide receivers making highlight reel grabs on ESPN.

My grandmother told me, "God put you on this Earth to teach people how to be strong."

When I was 12 years old, I knew that my ankles would feel better if I moved them around before I went to sleep. I had this program I created where I would take them through all these flexing and circular motions, because I knew that would help them. I've been obsessed with using science to improve human performance since I was 12. And if I could fix that 12-year-old kid, I could help anyone.

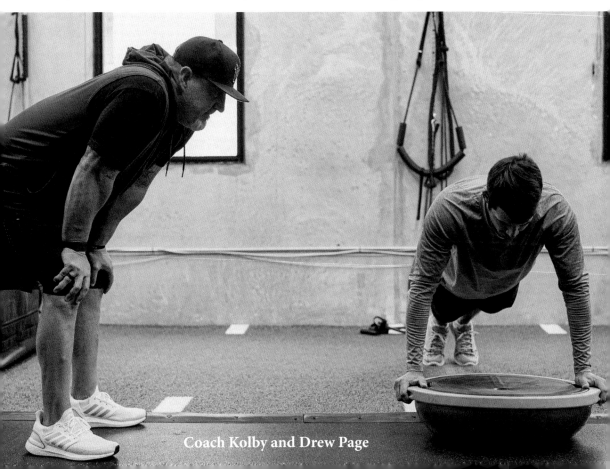

Coach Kolby and Drew Page

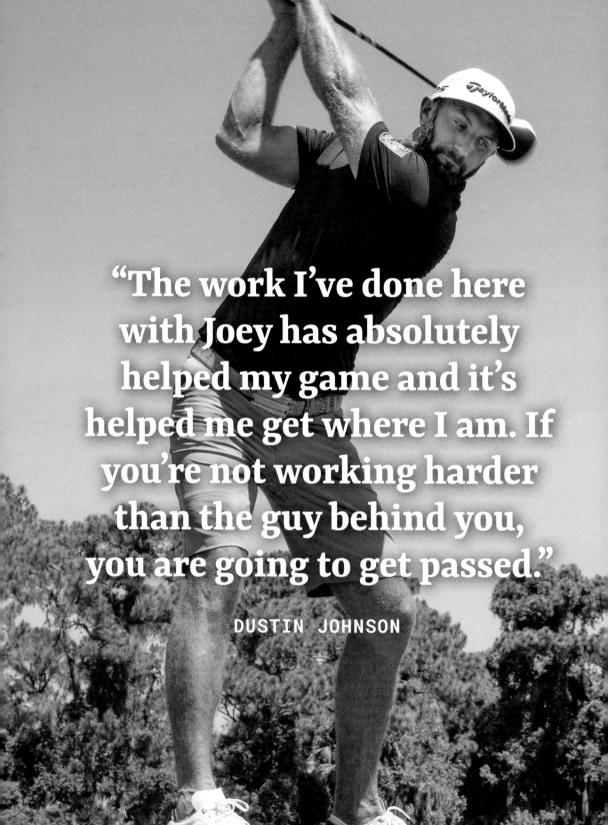

"The work I've done here with Joey has absolutely helped my game and it's helped me get where I am. If you're not working harder than the guy behind you, you are going to get passed."

DUSTIN JOHNSON

Species-Specific before Sports-Specific

You are a lion. You're the king of beasts. All other creatures fear and respect you.

Sort of.

Have you ever gone to the zoo and stopped by where they keep the lions? You see these massive and powerful animals strutting around. Every once in a while, one might let out a growl that starts out so deep and resonant that you'd think it was coming from the Earth's core. A few minutes later, someone from the zoo tosses it a huge chunk of meat and it inhales it while resting in the shade. Then it might take a nap.

Yes, this is a lion. If you were a geneticist and did a series of tests on the animal, all the results would come back reading, "Lion." But how would this country club lion fare if you dropped it into the heart of the Serengeti? It would probably get its lunch eaten – and probably a lot more – by the first pack of hyaenas it came up against. Why? Because lions were designed to hunt, stalk, run, jump, and kill. The lion in the zoo doesn't have to do any of this. The zoo is a combination of a prison and a high-end assisted-living facility. You're not free to leave, but it ain't such a bad gig overall. As a result of this lifestyle, though, the lion loses all the skills, movement patterns, neurological fine-tuning, and musculature that really defines what makes a lion a lion.

(Sure, it may have to defend its prime spot in the shade from other lions, but all that's proving is that it's the toughest of a bunch of de-toughened lions.)

So, getting back to the opening line of the chapter, you ARE a lion; you're just not quite the type of lion you think you are.

Just like the lion whose DNA tells it that it needs to run, jump, spot things moving hundreds of yards away, etc., you – as a human – have a genetic code that would have you being able to do all sorts of things that you don't actually do in real life. And, as people, we've had a far bigger head start than zoo animals when it comes to distancing ourselves and our bodies from what we and our bodies were designed to do. Humans in their latest form have been wandering around for about 100,000 years. And in that time, we've gone from being active hunters and gatherers to being sedentary accountants and programmers.

So, what can we do about it?

Before you can even think about taking your training in a sport-specific direction, you first need to focus on species-specific training. You need to be able to move your body the way human beings were intended to move and how our oldest ancestors moved their bodies. If your body is optimized to move as a human, you're now a blank canvas. And on that blank canvas, you can now paint yourself as a golfer, javelin thrower, tennis player, whatever.

But while an artist can just whitewash over an old painting to be able to start with a fresh canvas, things aren't quite as easy when it comes to the human body.

Undoing 5, 10, or 40 years of incorrect movement patterns doesn't happen overnight, but it can happen. If you've been playing reasonably well and haven't been doing the things necessary to change your body – and these changes are both physical and neurological – you've been having success with about half of your total potential. You're playing well despite yourself. The main thing that's getting in the way of you improving is your own body. Your mistakes out on the course are really about you not being able to get out of your own way. (And there are guys right now on the PGA Tour that would fall into this category!) But if you can get your feet to connect firmly with the ground regardless of your lie, if you can get your shoulders to externally rotate properly and with ease, and if you can accelerate explosively and decelerate comfortably and with control, these are game changers.

And while a lot of these things can be partially achieved by making your body physically stronger, you're not going to completely achieve them without making your body more neurologically efficient. It's about activating and engaging the muscles specific for creating and controlling the perfect golf swing. It's this neurological side of the training that's the least understood by people. You see it all the time. Guys at the course get ready to hit a golf ball by going out and hitting golf balls. You don't get ready to hit a golf ball by hitting golf balls; you need to first get your body ready to go swing a golf club. When your body has been properly neurologically activated and physically prepared to swing a club properly, then it's time to hit some balls. It's a process.

> *"Working out has always been a part of my job and I love it. To play at the highest level, it's a non-negotiable part of my daily training program. But some days it's easier said than done. Joey D can be a bear of a task master when he needs to be. For me, I like that. I perform best when I'm challenged – especially when it's someone I respect."* – **Brooks Koepka**

Your nervous system is made up of your brain, spinal cord, and pathways of nerves that reach out to every muscle in the body. Your brain is like the computer that's running the whole show, and the spinal cord and nerves are like the wires that transmit information to and from this computer to your body's "peripherals." In this case, the peripherals aren't printers, monitors, and speakers. The hardware in this case is your arms, legs, and the rest of the muscles of the body.

A lot of the things the nervous system is responsible for are done automatically, without you really having to think about them – breathing, digestion, the beating of your heart, etc. Other things have to be learned and improved through training. You can think of the training you do as being like updating your body's own software.

A quick example of neuromuscular training: It's relatively easy for most people to stand on two feet. You can probably do it for a pretty long time without putting much thought into it. Think about the last time you had to wait in a long, snaking line at the airport or to get your driver's license renewed. Yes, it was a total drag, but at any point were you worried that you would topple over? Probably not.

Now, take that standing position and do it on one leg. It gets a little more challenging. Now, while standing on one leg, close your eyes. All of a sudden, things get a whole lot more difficult. Now, imagine being on one foot with your eyes closed – and doing it all on a balance pad or some other unstable surface. It gets even more challenging. Every time you add another level of confusion and chaos to this one-legged progression, you attack your neurological system a little bit more.

The fun part is that over time, what once seemed like an impossible feat of balance and stability becomes a lot easier to do. Your brain is being trained to become even more of a supercomputer than it already was, and it can now process the millions of calculations required to keep you upright under a variety of different conditions and stressors.

Balancing on an unstable surface is one thing – and a good thing! – but think about trying to create power and movement on the same unstable surface using resistance bands, weights, or simply your own body. It'll improve the way you walk. It'll improve the way you run. It'll improve the way you hit a golf ball. And that supercomputer inside your head gets even more powerful. These are the vital neuromuscular adaptations that will make you a more effective human. And, in turn, will make you a better golfer.

> *"I've always been strong, but now I'm more athletic. My body just learned how to work better. What I always tell people is that what I'm doing in the gym attacks my neurological system. Previously, everything was just out of whack."*
> **– Talor Gooch**

And while getting your body's software as golf-ready as possible is important, no less important is getting your body's hardware just as golf-ready. And that's where heavier resistance training comes in.

Just because you see a golfer lifting weights, it doesn't mean he or she is going to become a bodybuilder. As long as the body maintains its golf-functionality and ranges of motion, more muscle isn't going to negatively affect your game.

Look at Brooks Koepka. He's the poster child of what everyone used to say was the exact opposite of the way a golfer should train and look. He lifts heavy when he wants to and fills out a shirt like no golfer before him. Oh, and he's a machine on the course. As of this writing, he's won four of the last 12 majors he's played in and finished in the top 10 in five of the rest.

In reality, the easiest thing to do in the fitness world is to build muscle. You challenge the targeted muscle with progressively greater challenges over time and as long as you're feeding your body with the proper nutrition, the muscle will grow.

That said, one of the hardest things to do in the fitness world is to build muscles in a balanced and functional way to optimize the body for a specific sport or action. And that's what we do down here in Jupiter on a daily basis. It's not simply mindless squats, curls, and deadlifts. Everything has to have a purpose in the gym.

What people don't realize is all the other work that someone like a Brooks Koepka is doing behind the scenes. Sure, the golf magazines and the Internet like to play up the fact that he can throw some serious weight around, but the other things that he's doing to maintain the mobility, stability, and strength around his joints are what's truly letting him play at such an elite level. His size and musculature is going to let him move the club at a pretty fast pace, but if he can't maintain his balance throughout that swing and if he can't decelerate properly, he's not playing late into Sunday every time you watch a major. And he's probably going to get injured.

On the other end of the physical spectrum is Justin Thomas. When he started here, he had power, but we wanted to give his body the strength to handle that power. We needed to get his body strong and stable enough to handle his swing. He went from 147 pounds to 165 pounds and went from being number twenty-two in the world to being number one. But even at 165 pounds, he has to go out week after week and compete with guys that outweigh him by 30 or 40 pounds. There are no weight classes in golf; he's still a middleweight fighting against heavyweights. For him to play as well as he does, he has to get the absolute most out of his body and that's only going to happen by training both his body's hardware and software optimally for playing golf and staying healthy.

The ultimate goal is to have the risk of injury go down and the level of athletic performance go up. As far as the pros go, if they're playing golf, they're making money. If they're on the sidelines, no one is making any money. Your livelihood probably doesn't depend on your ability to play golf, but if golf is that one thing that you look forward to, that one thing that you've invested a lot of time and a lot of money in, you want to be able to play well. And if you're injured, you're not playing.

"Before, I didn't work out that much. I would do a little bit, but that was because I was either forced to or because I felt I had to, and I wasn't consistent with it. And now, it's just become a part of my life, and I really do love working out and I enjoy the grind." – **Justin Thomas**

When you're playing golf, you want to have the luxury of only having to think about playing golf. If you're standing at address and instead of thinking about distance and wind direction, your mind is off fretting about posture, spine angle, how tight your hamstrings are feeling, then you're already playing at a disadvantage. You're distracted. As we mentioned earlier, you're getting in the way of yourself. Compare the way you feel when the car you're driving is working perfectly to how you feel when the "Tire Pressure" or "Check Engine" light comes on. It's the same thing. Golf is enough of a test of nerves as it is. There's no upside to adding more things to worry about.

To play with as much peace of mind as possible, you have to have absolute confidence in your body's ability to swing a club correctly. We've already stressed the importance of species-specific training and of the training of both your hardware and your software – your muscular system and your nervous system. Now, let's get sport-specific and look at just what your body has to do to swing a club – and why neuromuscular training is so important. And for that, we're going to introduce another system – the skeletal system.

Biomechanics is the study of how external forces – gravity, momentum, your muscles – affect the skeletal system. The golf swing can either be a beautiful symphony of gravity, momentum, and muscle working together to allow your skeletal system to drive a golf ball 300-plus yards or it can be a chaotic dirge of dysfunction that ends up with your ball hooking, slicing, popping straight up, or disappearing into any number of the hazards you were trying so hard to avoid.

For the most part, we're born with a relatively neutral skeletal system. At birth, you haven't yet spent 30 years hunched over a keyboard, sitting at a desk for eight hours at a clip, or doing hundreds of bench presses and other chest exercises at the gym without really focusing a whole lot on the muscles of the back. We're born with a straight spine and proper posture that hasn't been affected yet by your choice to become either a cell phone addict or a championship limbo dancer. It's everything you do from the moment you start crawling on the floor as a baby that begins to influence how your body will develop and – eventually – how you'll swing a golf club.

Most fitness and exercise books focus primarily on the muscles. If you want to look better in short sleeves, you flip over to the "Arms" chapter and you're given a bunch of variations on a biceps curl. You grab some dumbbells and start cranking out curls. Your biceps start to grow and you're feeling pretty good about life. The book also has a bunch of triceps exercise that work the back of the upper arm, but they're slightly more contrived then the biceps curl. The positions you need to be in aren't as simple as just standing and doing curls, and when you look in the mirror, the triceps exercises don't seem to give you that fast pump of instant gratification that curls do. So, what do most folks do? They focus primarily on the biceps exercises and neglect the triceps exercises.

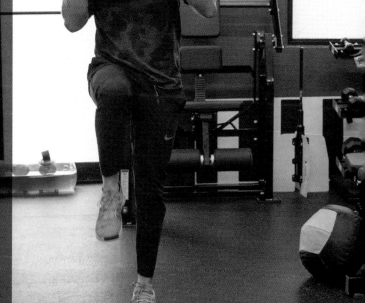

"I've always been strong, but now I'm more athletic. My body just learned how to work better. What I'm doing in the gym attacks my neurological system. Previously, everything was just out of whack."

TALOR GOOCH

The job of the muscle is to create movement around a joint. The job of your biceps, for example, is to bend your elbow. Curls do a really good job of isolating the biceps. The larger and stronger your biceps become, the greater the amount of force you will be able to generate by bending your elbow and the more weight you'll be able to curl.

And here's where the problems start.

The major joints of the body have pairs of muscles that work in partnership to create opposing movements around the joint. While the job of the biceps is to flex the arm at the elbow, the job of the triceps is to straighten the arm at the elbow. So if you're in the gym focusing almost exclusively on your biceps while ignoring your triceps, you may think you're doing great things for your body – heck, you look pretty damn good in the mirror! – but in reality you're creating dysfunction. Your biceps are now in a chronically shortened or tight position, while your triceps are now in a chronically lengthened position. Or, to create a visual, you're no longer able to completely straighten your arm. And while this isn't a life-threatening condition,

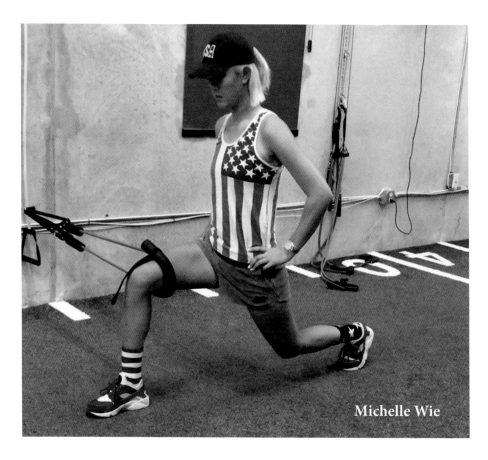

Michelle Wie

this imbalance around the elbow joint can create dysfunction that will affect your golf swing.

If you aren't able to straighten your arms during your golf swing, you'll have a tendency to get into a "chicken wing" scenario in either your takeaway or follow-through – or both – which will take you out of a proper swing plane and will affect your accuracy and power. You're also shortening the combined length of your arms and your club. Again, more loss of power and distance. Physics 101 tells us that the longer the length of your arms and the club is, the more speed you'll be able to generate at impact.

And that's just looking at potential dysfunction at the elbow, which is one of the simpler joints of the body. Think about all the ways that the arm can move at the shoulder or all the ways the leg can move at the hip. And for every one of those movements, there are muscles that are responsible for creating that movement and muscles responsible for creating an opposing movement. If you're focusing solely on the muscles and not how they impact proper movement around the joint, you may end up looking good, but you're not going to be playing at anywhere near your potential.

Dysfunction at a joint can not only cause issues at that particular joint, but it can also affect neighboring joints. As you'll see, dysfunction at the knee can affect hip movement, and problems at the elbow can lead to wrist issues. And in extreme cases, dysfunction in one place can lead to dysfunction in some distant and unlikely places.

"I was having wrist issues. I was using my wrists too much because my thoracic spine wasn't moving and I was really stiff in my upper back. So, because I wasn't following through with my body, I was compensating with my wrists to get the club through. We worked on getting my mobility back, so I could end up generating more power from the bigger muscles of the back and core instead of the smaller muscles at the wrist. I started working with Kolby at the end of 2017 and won my first tournament since 2014 in early 2018, so I think that shows how good he is." – **Michelle Wie**

The next eight chapters will focus on the major joints and skeletal structures of the body – from the ground up, starting with the feet and ankles, where the golf swing begins, up through the knees and into the hips, where the majority of your power is generated. We'll look at all of the things that can affect proper posture at the spine and at the neck and head. We'll address proper internal and external rotation at the shoulders and then go down the arm to the elbow and, finally, into the wrists and hands, where your connection with your club is your body's final chance to influence your swing.

We'll explain the function of each joint from an anatomical viewpoint and then address its role in the golf swing and what can happen if there's dysfunction at the joint. For each joint or structure, we'll provide three types of exercises – mobility movements, stability movements, and strength movements – to ensure that you're creating function and not dysfunction. We've even included modifications for some of the movements to make sure that there's a version you can do regardless of your current level of fitness or conditioning. And we've provided progressions for many of the movements so that you can move on to a more challenging version of the exercise as your body becomes stronger and more stable.

> *"After the first couple of workouts, I was just blown away by how much work I had to do, but also amazed at how much I enjoyed the workouts and how knowledgeable Kolby was. It was so different from coming from a college workout system, where you're typically stuck with the football meathead trainer and you're not really doing a functional workout program for a golfer."*
> **– Smylie Kaufman**

The goal of this book is to make you a better golfer. Plain and simple. But unless you're playing on one of the pro tours, you probably don't have hours every day to improve your game. We respect your time and, for that reason, have broken the program down into ever-changing half-hour workouts that you'll do three times a week. We don't think 90 minutes a week is too much to ask for in return for the improvements you'll see and feel after just a few workouts. The ever-changing workouts will not only keep things more interesting for you, but by switching up the exercises on a regular basis, we'll also continue our plan of keeping your neurological system continually challenged.

We also understand that golf is expensive, but we know that training the body properly doesn't have to be. We're not asking you to invest in a gym membership or hundreds of dollars' worth of equipment to make the most out of this program. It's all done with simple and inexpensive tools that won't set you back too much - resistance bands, balance pods, furniture sliders, a stability ball, and some light dumbbells are all you need.

> *"If I go somewhere and the hotel doesn't have a good gym, Kolby's basically able to make a workout out of nothing. Sometimes, I'll admit to him 'I didn't bring any of my bands and I don't have a gym, so what can I do?' And five minutes later, he'll shoot over some workout that's quite intense and quite challenging and all I've used for equipment is like a pillow or something."* – **Ben Taylor**

Get ready to shoot lower scores, have more fun out on the course, and become the golfer you always knew you could be.

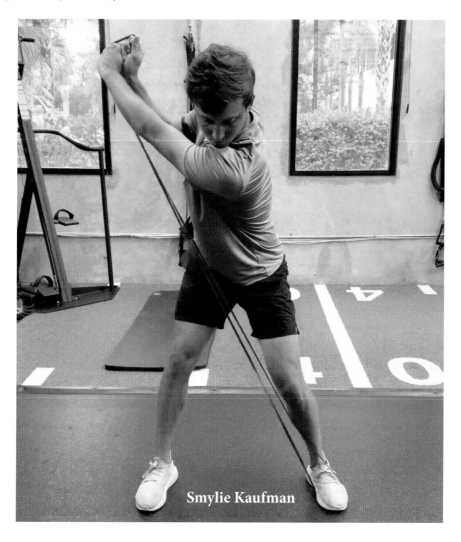

Smylie Kaufman

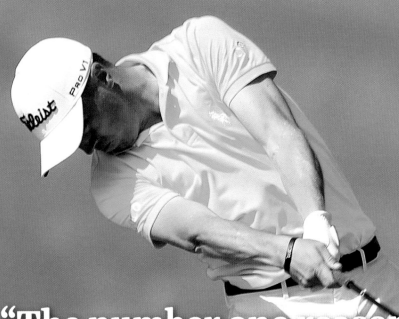

"The number one reason we're training and spending all that time in the gym is to get stronger and to avoid injuries. If we can get stronger, more mobile, and functional, then we win all around."

JUSTIN THOMAS

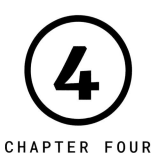

CHAPTER FOUR

The Ankle & Foot

While the ankle may not be the first body part that comes to mind when you think about athletic performance, it's the only one that's become part of mythology. You've heard of Achilles' heel; you've never heard of Apollo's hypermobile shoulder or Agamemnon's frayed meniscus.

From the waist down, the human skeletal system is pretty simple – until you get to the ankle. You have the femur, which is the sole bone of the thigh, the kneecap, and then the tibia and fibula, which are the two bones that make up the lower leg. It's a simple setup.

Then you get to the foot. There are 26 bones that make up the foot. That's right; you have 26 bones in each of your FootJoys. When you consider that an adult human has 206 total bones, it's fascinating that about a quarter of them are in your socks. And each of those bones has a job to do. On the plus side, having this many moving parts lets the foot do some amazing things. On the negative side, with this many parts, there's a lot of potential for injuries, imbalances, compensations, and dysfunctions.

For most people, having issues with any of the bones that make up the foot and ankle isn't necessarily a deal-breaker. If you've ever stubbed your toe – and probably caused a slight fracture – you may limp for a few days, but your life won't be significantly impacted. The same thing holds true if you've ever rolled your ankle. There might be swelling and some temporary changes to the way you walk, but you can still go to work and you can still be a functional member of society.

If you're a golfer, though, either of these situations – plus any number of other dysfunctions involving the foot and ankle – can powerfully affect your golf game.

The Primary Movement of the Ankle & Foot

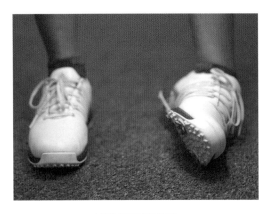

INVERSION

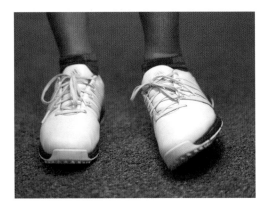

EVERSION

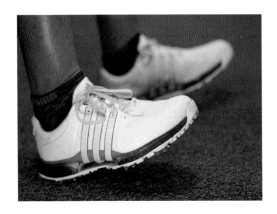

DORSIFLEXION

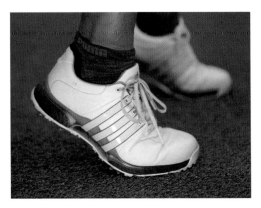

PLANTARFLEXION

And not in a positive way. Players are always surprised at how much attention and focus we put on the ankle, but golf is a game played on two feet, so if you're not looking at how to improve the way your feet connect with the ground, you're missing a vital way to improve your game. It would be like deciding not to work on your short game.

Before we think about ways to keep your ankles mobile, stable, and strong, let's take a look at how the ankle and foot move and what has to happen every time you walk, run, or drive a golf ball.

The primary movements at the ankle are plantarflexion, dorsiflexion, inversion, and eversion. It sounds more complicated than it is. Think about the angle of your lower leg and foot at the ankle when you're just standing up straight. It's 90 degrees. Plantarflexion at the ankle just means that you can push down with the ball of your foot like you're stepping on the gas pedal. In this case, the angle of your lower leg and foot is now greater than 90 degrees. Dorsiflexion is the opposite motion. Imagine lifting the ball of your foot and toes off the ground while keeping your heel on the ground. Now that same angle is less than 90 degrees.

Inversion is a sideways motion where you ride the outer edge of the foot and the inner edge of the foot comes off the ground. (Inversion, at its most extreme, is how people roll their ankles.) Eversion is the opposite motion. It's a sideways motion where your weight goes into the inner edge of the foot and the outer edge comes off the ground. (Remember, the human body is all about opposing movements.)

To be able to perform all of these movements with as much control and balance as possible on both flat and unstable or irregular surfaces, the bones of the mid foot and toes are called in to help with mobility and stability. And that's why a quarter of your bones are in your feet!

The Ankle & Foot

A DETAIL OF THE JOINT, MUSCLES, AND TENDONS

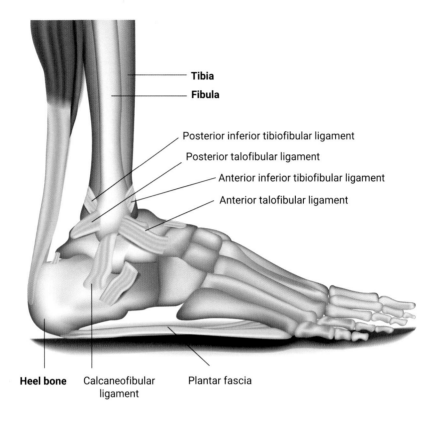

Tibia

Fibula

Posterior inferior tibiofibular ligament

Posterior talofibular ligament

Anterior inferior tibiofibular ligament

Anterior talofibular ligament

Heel bone   Calcaneofibular
ligament

Plantar fascia

On the golf course, your body needs to be able to take advantage of all four of these major movements at the ankle to optimally hit the ball. The ankles and feet are the foundation of the golf swing. They're what's holding up the building. Without proper stability and control, this becomes a very weak foundation.

At address, your knees are slightly bent, which means the angle of your foot and lower leg is less than 90 degrees. If you don't have the mobility to get into this position, it means you'll be playing from a more straight-legged setup. Generally, this will result in a very arms-y swing. When we see an upper body dominant player, the first thing we look at is what the feet are doing.

As you go into your takeaway and backswing, there's a lot of momentum riding into your back foot. If you don't have the strength around the ankle to resist this force, your ankle will begin to roll and the inner edge of the foot will lose contact with the ground. Once this happens, you've already begun to lose your balance. Trying to recover your balance mid-swing is never a good thing to have to do. Your timing is thrown off, and both power and accuracy will suffer.

As you begin your downswing, your balance is now shifting forward toward your target, and you need to be able to evert your back foot – load into the inner edge of the foot. If you don't have the strength and mobility to do this, even if everything else was perfect up this point, you'll end up flat-footed and have a weakened upper-body-dominant shot.

Finally, as your hips turn through impact, power is generated by pushing into the ground with the ball of your foot and plantarflexing the back foot. If there's not sufficient strength, power will suffer greatly.

And that's just your back foot!

Your front foot has to withstand the giant back-and-forth shift in momentum from takeaway into downswing and impact and not lose its connection with the ground.

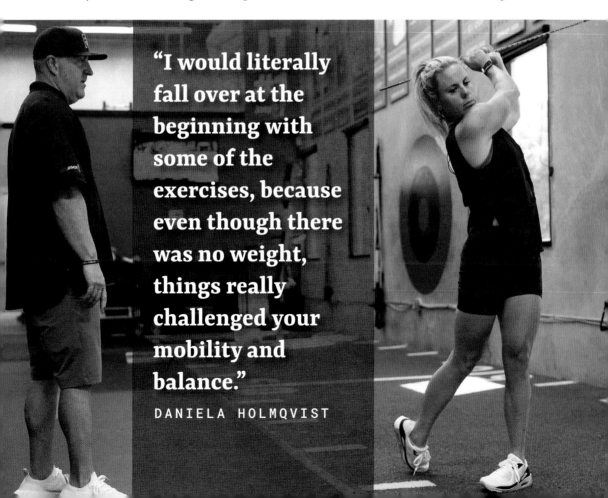

"I would literally fall over at the beginning with some of the exercises, because even though there was no weight, things really challenged your mobility and balance."

DANIELA HOLMQVIST

A Delicate Balancing Act

Balance is one of the least understood aspects of sports performance. But what exactly is it? How does it work? And can balance be improved?

Most people assume that balance is like height. You get whatever your DNA says you're supposed to get.

Balance is actually a combination of three different things. A lot of it has to do with vision. We're better able to stay upright and move in a controlled way with our eyes open. If we're able to anchor ourselves visually to something nonmoving, it lets us control our own movement more precisely.

The second element is the series of liquid-filled canals in our inner ears that act like gyroscopes to keep us oriented in space. Want to mess with those gyroscopes to see what happens? Stand in the middle of a room with plenty of free space around you. Now start spinning around. The faster and longer you spin, the more disoriented – or dizzy – you'll become. (And if you want to see how really important vision is to balance, close your eyes after you're done spinning!) Eventually, as the liquid in our gyroscopes settles, the world gets back to normal.

Finally, the nervous system plays a key part in keeping you upright and stable. One of the jobs of our body's "software" is to keep us from falling down. As we discussed in Chapter 3, by challenging the neuromuscular system, we're able to improve balance. And, of the three balance components, this is the one we have most control over.

That's important. As we age, our vision is going to deteriorate slightly and the fluid-filled canals in the inner ear can get damaged, infected, and lose their efficiency. To help prevent potential issues down the road – and to make you a better golfer right now – working on balance is a must.

And while all these scenarios are scary enough when you're just thinking about your tee shot, imagine the added requirements around the ankle when you've got an uphill lie, a downhill lie, or any number of other situations when you're not on a completely flat surface. You're only guaranteed 18 shots per round off a flat, even surface.

And sometimes, you're not even guaranteed a solid surface to hit from. From the outside looking in, people often wonder why a lot of the things we do in the gym are on unstable surfaces like balance pads. They'll say things like, "Why do things on a balance pad when I'm going to be swinging standing on the ground? The ground doesn't move." You ever hit out of a bunker? You ever hit after a rain delay? Guess what? The ground moves.

Look at what Dustin Johnson had to deal with in a span of minutes on the 15th hole of the 2020 Travelers Championship. Up by two strokes, his drive on the par 4 came within inches of landing in the water. With no other option, he took off his shoes and socks, rolled up his pants, and hit the ball while standing ankle deep in water. His next shot – with shoes and socks back on – was from an uneven lie in the heavy rough. A minute later, he's knocking in a four-foot putt to par the hole and maintain his two-stroke lead. He went on to win by a single stroke. For his ability to handle all

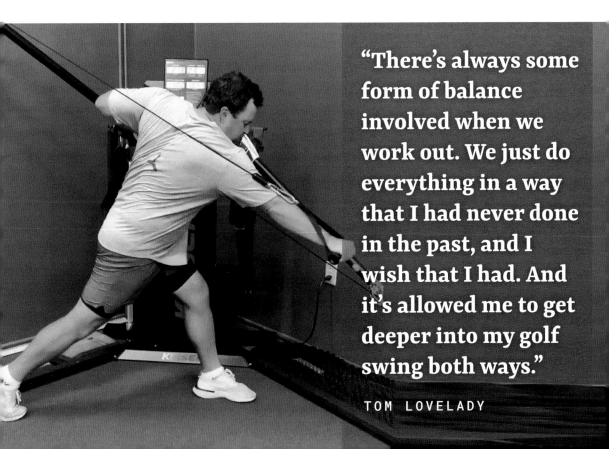

"There's always some form of balance involved when we work out. We just do everything in a way that I had never done in the past, and I wish that I had. And it's allowed me to get deeper into my golf swing both ways."

TOM LOVELADY

that the Golf Gods could throw at him, Dustin increased his stretch of consecutive years with a Tour victory to a daunting 13.

That's why we train on unstable surfaces!

With all this riding on your ankles, it's important to keep the muscles that operate around the joint strong and in balance with each other. The biggest muscle of the lower leg is maybe the one that most people have heard of. The gastrocnemius is the primary muscle that plantarflexes the foot. It's the stepping on the gas muscle. It's the far biggest for a reason. Every step you take forces the gastrocnemius into action. When someone has large, well-developed calves, it's the gastrocnemius that you're seeing. The other muscles that work around the joint are more about stability than strength, which is why they're not as large. And it's also why you've probably never heard of them. It's not important that you know or memorize their names. What is important is that you realize that you have essentially four muscles that are responsible for the four major movements of the ankle.

The anterior tibialis moves the ankle in the opposite direction than the gastrocnemius. It pulls the toes up as opposed to pushing them down. The peroneals are along the outer side of the lower leg. When they contract or shorten, the outer edge of the foot lifts. They are the muscles that help stabilize the foot during your takeaway and help give you power through impact. The posterior tibialis, along the inside of your lower leg, works with the peroneals to assist in side-to-side ankle stabilization.

One of the main goals of having all of these muscles optimally tuned and working together is that these are the muscles primarily responsible for balance. And once you start doing some of the balance-based exercises in this book, you'll really begin to have new awareness of – and appreciation for – everything that takes place around the ankle joint.

In addition to the mobility, stability, and strength exercises that we're about to show you, there are some other considerations to think about when it comes to the foot and ankle.

You also have to look at what you're wearing on your feet, which is why shoe companies have thrown so much into research and development in shoe design. It's not enough to choose a shoe just because they look good with your favorite pants or they're the same style that your favorite pro wears. Shoes need to not only offer maximum support where stability is needed, but also allow for maximum freedom where mobility is needed. It's important that, in a shoe, the foot can, as much as possible, feel what it needs to be able to feel in terms of connecting with the ground.

Another important thing to think about is the shoes that you wear when you're NOT golfing. If you're wearing a boot that has a heel or if you're someone who wears a lot of high-heeled shoes, you may be sacrificing your golf game in exchange for a couple extra inches of height or the appearance of sexier calves. Heeled shoes put your ankle into plantarflexion, which means that the muscles of the calf are constantly engaged, shortened, and tightened. In short, your calf is like a clenched fist. Over time, this can greatly affect your ankles' ability to dorsiflex properly. As we just talked about, dorsiflexion is the ankles' starting point at address. If your address position is overly straight-legged because of the lack of mobility at the ankle, again, your swing may be doomed even before you've gone into your backswing.

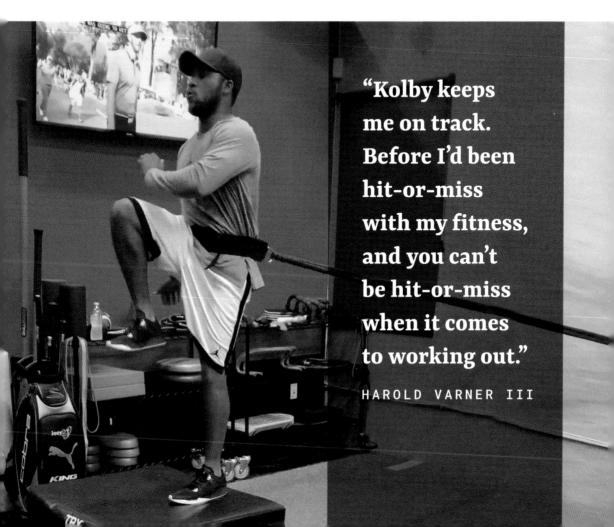

"Kolby keeps me on track. Before I'd been hit-or-miss with my fitness, and you can't be hit-or-miss when it comes to working out."

HAROLD VARNER III

Golf Ball Foot Hurdles

ANKLE & FOOT MOBILITY

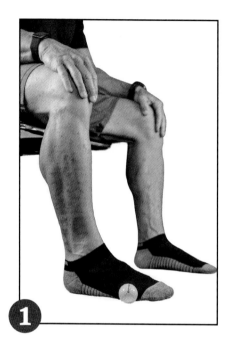
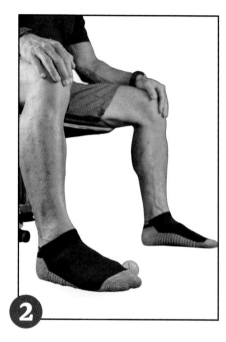

1) Sit on a bench or chair in an upright position with feet flat on the floor. Place a golf ball on the floor just to the right of your right baby toe.

2) Keeping your heel on the floor, lift the ball of your foot and toes off the floor and pass it over the ball. When you put your foot down, the ball should now be just to the left of your big toe. Do 10 "hurdles" over the ball and then switch to the left foot. The key to the move is not lifting the heel off the floor. Do three sets of 10 with each foot.

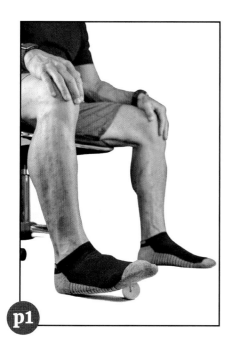 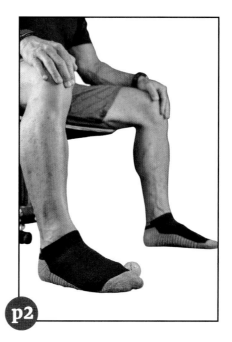

Progression One: To further increase mobility around the ankle, do the same movement, but this time when you do the initial movement with your right foot, only touch the outer edge of the foot to the floor. On the return hurdle, try to only touch the inner edge of the foot to the floor. Again, the heel should be in contact with the floor at all times. This is a very subtle variation of the initial movement, so take your time to get it right.

Progression Two: A little bit tougher than the first progression. This time, only touch the INNER edge of the foot to the floor on the initial outward hurdle. On the inward hurdles, try to only touch the OUTER edge of the foot to the floor. Again, shoot for three sets of 10 hurdles on each foot.

Single-Leg Standing Balance

ANKLE STABILITY

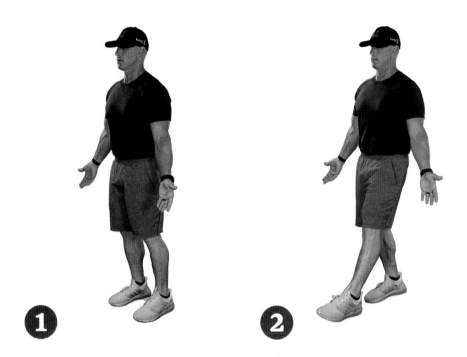

1) Stand in a comfortable stance with feet shoulder-width apart. Slowly shift your weight over your right leg and – keeping your left leg straight – slightly lift your left foot off the floor. This is the starting position.

2) Imagine that you're standing in the middle of a giant clockface. Keeping your left leg straight raise it in front of you (or where 12:00 would be on the clock). Hold this position for a two-count and then return to the starting position without touching the foot to the ground.

3) Now, lift it out to the side (or toward 9:00) and hold it for a two-count.

4) Return to the starting position again without touching the foot to the ground and now extend the leg in back of you (or toward 6:00). Hold this for a two-count and then return to the starting position. Switch feet and do the same series of movements with the left foot on the floor.

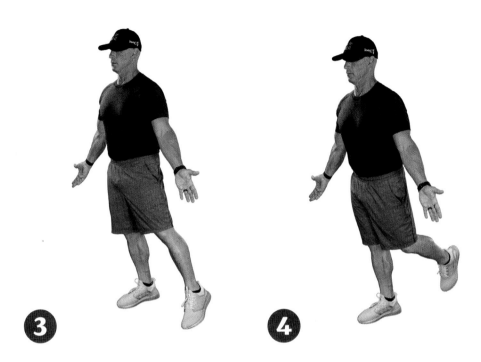

Initially, alternate between feet after only one set of the three moves. Work up to the point where you can do three complete sets of 12:00, 9:00 (or 3:00 with your right foot), and 6:00 on each side without putting the foot down before you switch feet.

Try this both barefoot and with shoes on. Being barefoot will give you more control over your balance, but since you play golf in shoes, it's important to be able to feel how balance works without as much connection with the ground. You may be surprised at how different things feel with and without shoes!

Progression One: Once you've mastered the movements on a stable surface, try doing them on a balance pad or balance disc.

Progression Two: Improve stability even more – and get in some bonus neuromuscular work – by trying the movements with your eyes closed. Start on a solid surface and work your way up to doing them on a balance pad or disc.

Standing Calf Raise

GASTROCNEMIUS STRENGTH AT THE ANKLE

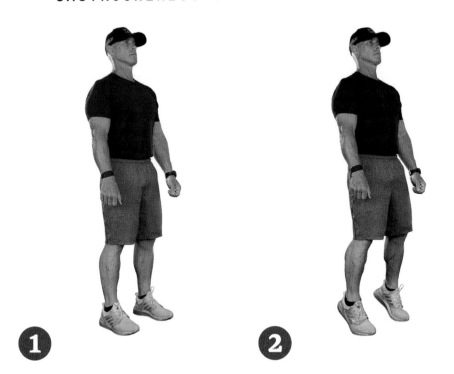

1) Stand with feet shoulder-width apart.

2) Come up as high as you can on your tiptoes, hold this position for a moment, and then slowly lower yourself almost back to the starting position but without quite touching your heels to the floor. Initially shoot for a set of 15 without touching your heels to the floor. Over time, keep increasing sets by five reps until you can do 30 raises relatively easily.

Progression One: Perform the same calf raises as above, but this time holding a 15- or 20-pound dumbbell in each hand. Start with sets of 10 and – over time – increase sets by two reps until you get to 20.

Progression Two: Stand with feet next to each other holding a dumbbell in each hand. (You can go with lighter dumbbells until you get a feel for the movement.) Raise your left knee up in front of you until your left thigh is parallel to the floor. Come up as high as you can on your tiptoes with your right foot, hold for a moment, and then lower yourself without quite letting your right heel touch the floor. Shoot for 10 on each leg without touching your heel to the floor.

Toe Raises

ANTERIOR TIBIALIS STRENGTH AT THE ANKLE

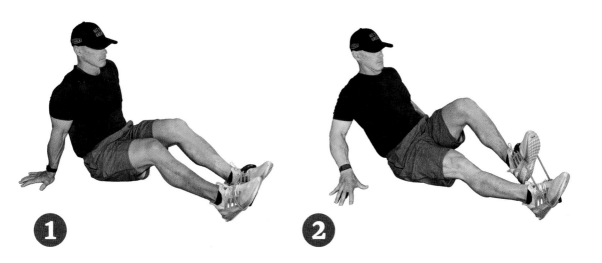

1) To target the muscle on the front of your lower leg, sit on the floor with a loop resistance band looped around both your feet. Half of the band will be under the soles of your feet and the other half will be on top of your feet and running over your shoelaces. Place your hands slightly behind and away from both hips.

2) Maintaining good upright posture, raise your left knee so your thigh is elevated 30 to 45 degrees from the floor. Establish solid balance in this position. You may be feeling some work going on in the front of your left hip. This is the starting position.

Slowly, while maintaining a good posture and without moving anything else, pull the toes of your left foot up as if you were trying to point them over your head. Your knee should remain bent. All the movement should happen at the ankle. Hold for three to five seconds at the highest point you can point them (and it won't actually be pointing over your head, trust us). Slowly, with movement only at the ankle, return to the starting position to complete the rep. This is a tough movement, so go slow and stay in control.

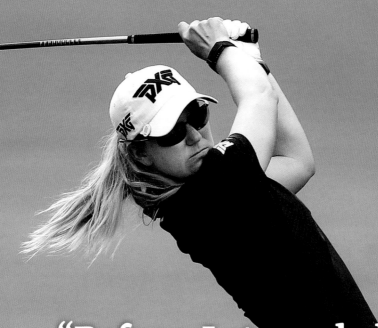

"Before, I struggled with pain at some point each season. Working with Kolby, I've never felt better."

AUSTIN ERNST

CHAPTER FIVE

The Knee

Knees and sports injuries, unfortunately, go together like Florida and sunshine. ACL tears, alone, have ended the careers of more athletes than you can probably remember. On the plus side, ACL tears are almost completely unheard of in golf. Golfers don't have to change direction while running at full speed, nor are they constantly getting their legs taken out from under them by aggressive defensive players. This, however, doesn't mean golfers don't have to worry about their knees when they play or train. Any number of dysfunctions around the knee joint can add strokes – and frustration – to your game.

While we've talked about all the different ways there can be movement around the ankle joint, movement around the knee joint is a lot simpler. There are only two movements that happen around the knee. The leg can bend (flexion) … or the leg can straighten (extension). The joint is like a hinge connecting a door to a door frame. The door can open and the door can close. That's it. If the door does anything else, it's because something has gone horribly wrong. Similarly, if you get any movement at the knee that isn't simply flexion and extension, something has gone horribly wrong – and you'll be in a world of pain.

> *"Coming back from my knee surgery, Joey not only knew what he could do to continue my overall progress, but he also worked closely with my doctor to make sure the knee rehab was done correctly."* – **Dustin Johnson**

Unlike the ankle, where we needed stability, mobility, and strength in roughly similar amounts for the golf swing, the requirement at the knee is primarily about stability. If the knee can be stabilized correctly, it'll make controlling the hips – the main lower-body power source for the golf swing – a whole lot easier. The knee has to be stable in order for the hips to be mobile.

And a stable knee isn't necessary just for optimal golf. Going back to our thoughts on species-specific training, a stable knee is the key to proper human movement. You can't generate any power from the ground up without the knees being stable. Instability at the knee will affect the way you walk, run, jump, etc. A little instability will negatively affect athletic performance. A lot of instability can potentially lead to all sorts of ankle, foot, and lower back problems.

That's not to say we don't need mobility and strength at the knee. Both do play a part in the golf swing.

Before we get golf-specific about the role of the knee in your swing, let's look at the anatomy of the knee joint.

The primary muscles that operate around the knee are the muscles of the thigh. The quadriceps in the front of the thigh is the group of four muscles that take the leg from a bent position to a straight position. If you're sitting down right now while reading this, straighten your right leg in front of you so that the entire leg is parallel to the floor. If you feel the muscles on the front of your right thigh, they should feel

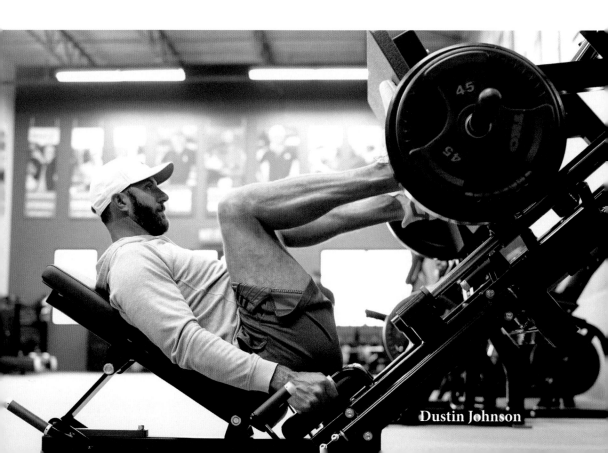

Dustin Johnson

The Anatomy of the Knee

A DETAIL OF THE JOINT AND MUSCLES

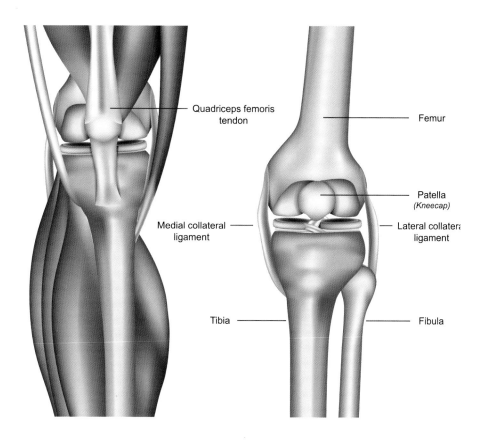

Quadriceps femoris tendon

Femur

Patella
(Kneecap)

Medial collateral ligament

Lateral collatera ligament

Tibia

Fibula

pretty solid and engaged. Now, feel the same muscles on the front of your left thigh. You're probably able to grab deeper into the muscle because it's relaxed and not engaged.

The group of three muscles on the back of the thigh – the hamstrings – are responsible for bending the leg at the knee. If you're a sports fan, you've probably heard and read far more about hamstring problems than quadriceps problems. Hamstring injuries due to overly tight muscles plague even elite athletes. If top-tier athletes, who have regimens and protocols for stretching, can have hamstring issues, it makes it all the more important for the casual athlete to pay attention to the backs of their thighs.

"I had some complications with my first knee surgery. Joey helped me come

back from that and it went great. I got a lot stronger." – **Steve Marino**

And it all goes back to our lion in the zoo. In a nutshell, we weren't meant as a species to sit so much. We sit on the way to work, we sit at work, we sit on the way home from work, we sit when we eat dinner, and then we sit while watching Golf Channel and ESPN. If our ancient ancestors sat around as much as we do today, we probably wouldn't be here today – mainly because they would have either starved to death or been eaten by predators. Unfortunately, sitting has become the human "default position." All that sitting puts the knee at a 90-degree angle a whole lot of the time and that means that the hamstrings are almost constantly in a shortened position. If we stood more, the hamstrings would be in a far less shortened position and in a far more neutral position for a lot longer time. And – as a result – our hamstrings wouldn't be so tight and susceptible to injury.

Tight hamstrings on the golf course won't necessarily lead to a hamstring pull, strain, or tear, but they will lead to other issues. Overly tight hamstrings will prevent you from maintaining proper golf posture throughout your swing and throughout your round. Tight hamstrings will prevent you from having optimal flexion – or bend – at the knees and hips. When this happens, players generally end up more straight-legged. And this leads to a rounded back as players try to figure out how to get low enough to hit the ball. A rounded back will lead to a very unpredictable swing plane, which hurts accuracy. Being overly straight-legged also takes a lot of movement and power production away from the hips, and this almost always results in a decrease in power and distance.

Creating the mobility to be able to maintain proper bend at the knee throughout the swing, though, isn't enough if there's a lack of stability around the joint. This is an issue that we see all the time. At takeaway, the front knee will buckle in slightly (or more than slightly) or the back knee will buckle out slightly. Either of these weaknesses will cause slight side-to-side shifts of the hips and take you out of proper swing plane. When we see this, we know that there are some muscular imbalances with the quadriceps on the front of the thigh. As the name implies, the quadriceps are made up of four muscles. When we see the inability to control side-to-side movement, we generally look at the innermost and outermost of these four muscles. (And if you want to get ultra-scientific about things, those muscles would be the vastus medialis on the inner side of the front of your thigh and the vastus lateralis on the outer side of the front of the thigh.) Engaging these muscles correctly will keep the knees stable and remove a couple of extra moving parts from your swing.

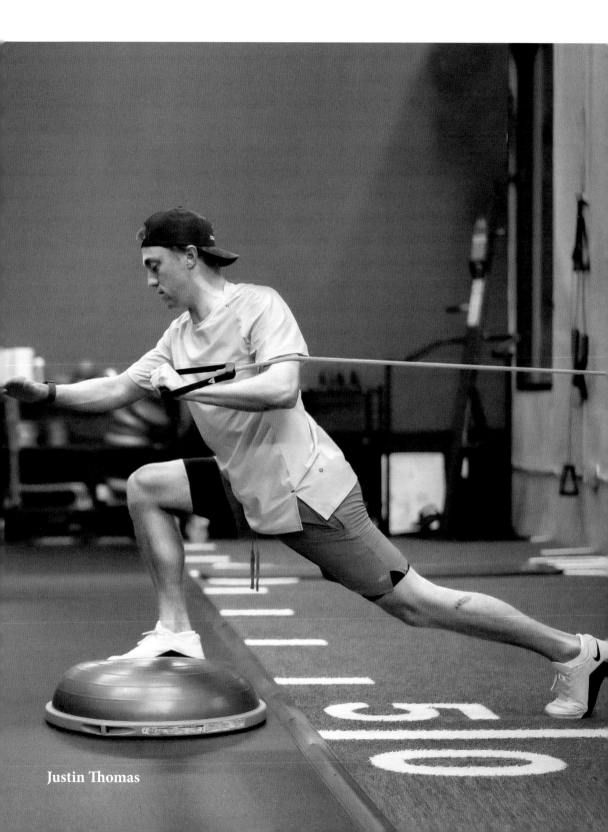

Justin Thomas

Sprains, Strains, Ligaments, Tendons & Muscles

As we discussed in Chapter 3, muscles are what move our bones and let us do everything from walking and putting food in our mouths to driving a golf ball. When muscles contract or shorten, they pull one bone closer to another and create movement. Muscles are fed through our cardiovascular system and because they can readily receive a steady supply of nutrients, muscles have the ability to heal themselves when injured. Depending on the degree of the tear or strain, even seemingly very nasty muscle pulls and injuries can heal on their own without surgery.

Tendons are the strong connective tissue that attaches muscle to bone. It's generally a lot stronger than the belly or body of the muscle it's a part of. Because they don't contract as much as muscle fiber, they don't receive the same amount of nutrients as muscle. This means that serious tendon strains or tears usually need some sort of surgical intervention to get things working properly again.

Ligaments are the strong fibrous tissue that connect bone directly to bone. They're sort of like the emergency brakes of the body. They're incredibly strong and it's their job to hold you together when your muscles can't. Because their role is more about stability than mobility, ligaments don't have the ability to shorten and lengthen as much as or as quickly as muscle. This means that if you roll your ankle and suffer a

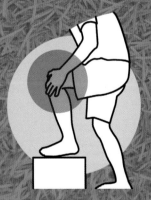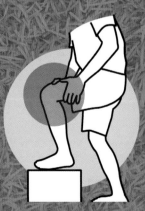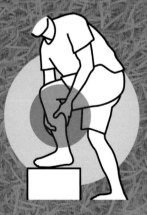

serious ligament sprain, you may be more likely in the future to suffer this same injury. (That's why it's so important to build up the muscle around a joint after an injury.)

A ligament tear is a much more serious situation. While muscle pulls and strains are the price we pay for being active human beings, ligament tears just aren't supposed to happen. And they usually take some serious force or trauma to occur. The most well-known ligament injury is an ACL (anterior cruciate ligament) tear. This is one of the ligaments that connects the femur – the main bone of the upper leg – to the tibia – one of the two bones that make up the lower leg. It plays a vital role in knee stability and when it gets damaged can result in a major lack of functionality at the knee. ACL tears almost always require surgical repair. Thankfully, golf doesn't require you to make lightning-quick direction changes while running, and very few golfers have ever had their legs taken out from under them by another golfer.

So, while an ACL tear shouldn't be high on your list of concerns out on the course, there are some things you want to be aware of. If you're a right-handed player, your swing – especially your follow-through – creates a lot of torque on your left knee. Finishing a 100-plus mph swing in classic position with your left foot still in essentially the same position it was at address, but with your hips turned toward your target, means that your left knee has to be able to withstand a good deal of very dynamic rotational force. That's why it's vital to work mobility, stability, and strength around the knee joint.

And if you were paying attention, you noticed that you strain a muscle or tendon, but you sprain a ligament.

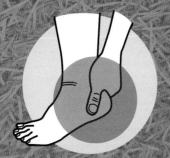 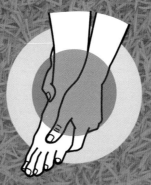 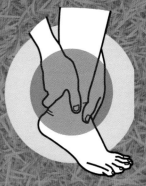

When mobility, stability, and strength are optimal, the knee becomes like a shock absorber that lets you adjust – up and down – to where you need to be throughout your swing. What we often see is that a player will want to generate as much speed and power as possible as he heads into his downswing. Instead of focusing on upper body movement to do this, he'll be like the guy at the carnival trying to ring the bell by using his entire body to slam downward with a sledgehammer. Yes, you will be able to generate power force by using a few more body parts, but the problem is that the goal of the golf swing isn't to ring a bell at the carnival by swinging a sledgehammer. Once you've done this and dropped your hips by bending at the knees, you've taken yourself out of an optimal swing plane.

If at setup your knees are bent at 130 degrees, it's important to have that same bend at the knee at impact if you want to be able to extend the arms and hit the ball with maximum power. If the knees are now more bent, though, the arm-club length needs to be shortened to make proper contact. The club isn't going to shorten itself on the fly, so what happens is that you have to bend the elbows slightly to compensate for the extra bend in the knees. You've shortened the striking lever in the equation and, as a result, you're sacrificing power. (You're also having to completely rethink and adjust your swing mid-swing! And that's never a good thing!) Think of the knees as being like hydraulics that lower and raise your body – and your center of gravity. If you can keep your hips at the proper height throughout your swing, you'll be able to have full arm extension – and maximum power – at impact.

One of the best ways to make sure that you'll have full extension at impact is to stabilize the knees and prevent unnecessary movement either up and down or from side to side. Going back to the sledgehammer at the carnival analogy, you will not be rewarded with a giant stuffed animal for taking yourself out of an optimal swing plane – no matter how much extra power you think it may give you.

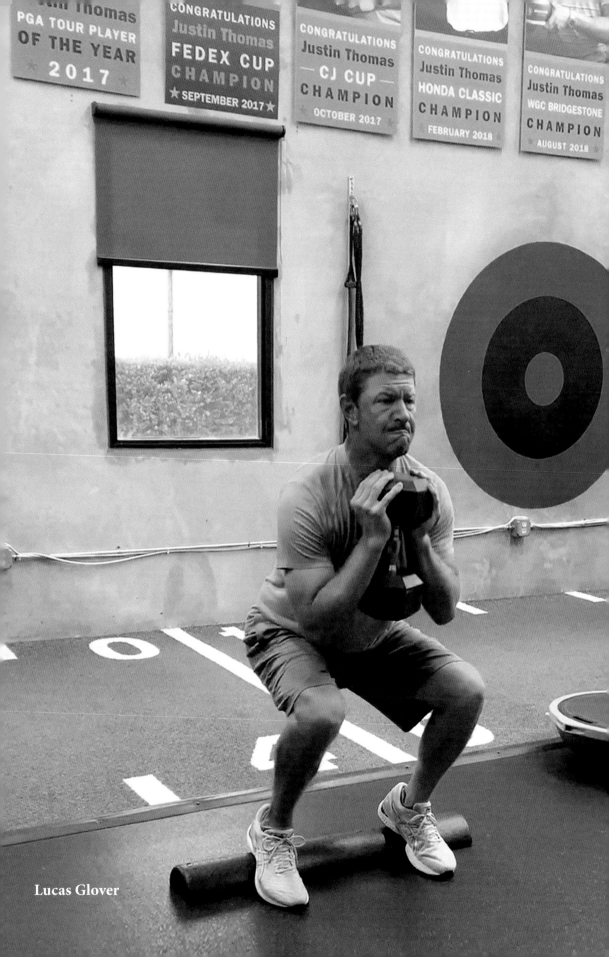

Lucas Glover

Romanian Deadlift

KNEE MOBILITY/HAMSTRING STRENGTH

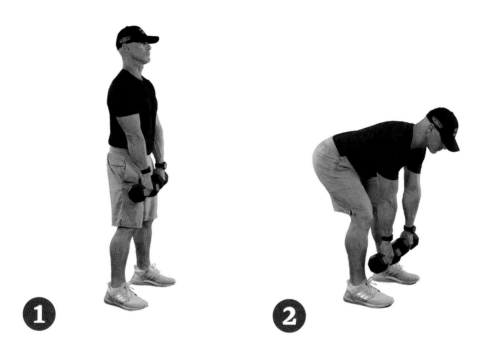

1) To keep the hamstrings in the back of your thighs loose – and to give them a strength challenge – stand straight-legged with feet shoulder-width apart and a light dumbbell in each hand. (As you get more efficient with the movement, you can add more weight.) The weights should be against the front of your thighs with your palms facing your thighs. This is the starting position.

2) While keeping the weights against your legs and your back straight, push your hips back and slowly lower the dumbbells. Your knees will bend slightly while you do this. When the dumbbells have gotten just below the knee, hold for a second, feel the stretch in the back of your thigh, and then push the hips forward, squeezing your glutes, and straightening your legs until you return to the starting position. Do 10 reps to complete the set.

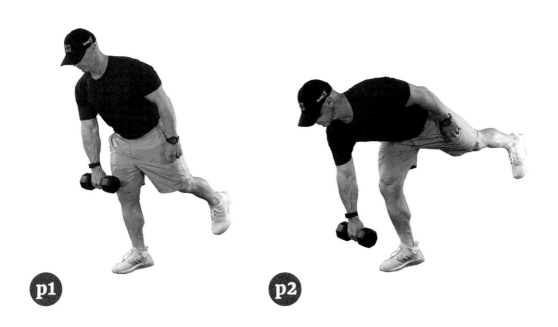

Progression One: Assume the same starting position as previously, but with your feet together and a dumbbell in your right hand only. As you begin to lower the weight against your leg, extend your left leg in back of you.

Progression Two: Your right leg will bend slightly, as above, but try to keep the left leg straight. Also try to keep your hips level. In other words, don't let your left hip raise higher than your right hip, which it will want to do. And don't let your left hip dip lower than your right hip, which it might also want to do. Picture one of those carpenter's leveling tools – the one with the bubble in it that moves when it's not on something flat – laying across your lower back and having the bubble staying firmly in the center. Establish your balance in this position and then slowly return to the starting position to complete the rep. Take your time with these to really fine-tune the movement. Work your way up to sets of 10 on each leg.

Lunges with Rotation

KNEE STABILITY

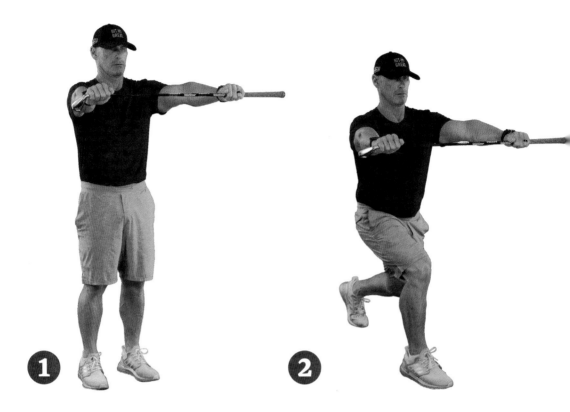

1) Stand with feet shoulder-width apart holding a club out in front of you horizontally at shoulder height. Your hands should be slightly wider than shoulder-width apart.

2) Take a deep step forward into a lunge position with your right leg. In the lunge position, your right knee should be directly over your right heel and your right knee should be bent to around 90 degrees. (Don't worry if you can't get your knee to 90 degrees if you're just starting out. That range of motion will eventually happen if you stick with it.) Your right knee shouldn't be caved in or bowed out to the side. It should be tracking right along the line of your second toe.

3) Maintaining a very upright posture, slowly rotate your upper body toward the right, keeping the club extended out in front of you at shoulder height. Make sure to turn your head as you turn your upper body. This will not only let you rotate a little deeper but will also challenge your balance more. Your right knee will want to bow

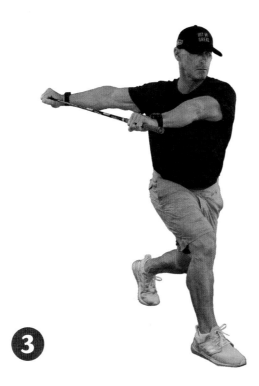

out a bit to the right when you do this, but try to keep it tracking over your second toe. Hold this position for a beat and then return to a forward-facing lunge position.

Reestablish your balance in the lunge position and then rotate your upper body to the left – or away from your lead leg. This time, your knee will want to follow your upper body and cave in to the left. Again, try not to let this happen. Hold this position for a beat, return to the forward-facing lunge position, reestablish your balance, and then, pushing off your right leg, return to the standing starting position. Now, step into a lunge with the left leg and do both rotations. Shoot for 10 lunges with rotations on each leg.

Progression: Perform the same movements holding a 55- or 65-centimeter stability ball instead of a golf club. This will add extra weight to the movement and the tweaked hand position and the way you're forced to hold the ball will add a chest-opening element to the exercise.

Split Lunge

QUADRICEPS STRENGTH AT THE KNEE

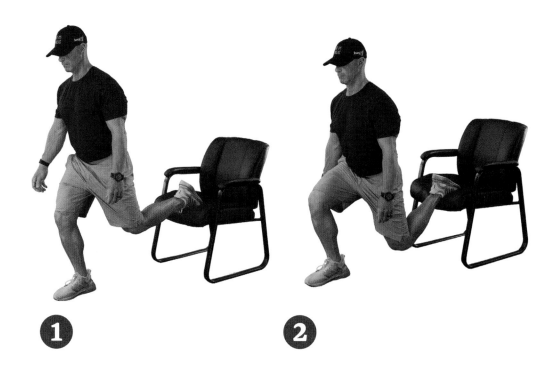

1) To build strength in the quadriceps, stand about two feet in front of a weight bench or anything else that's solid, stable, and stands about 18" to 24" off the floor. Carefully, extend your left leg in back of you and place your foot on the bench with your toes curled under. Hop forward or backward until your right knee is directly over your right heel. This is the starting position.

2) Keeping your right knee over your heel, slowly lower your hips until your knee is flexed to an angle smaller than 90 degrees. Hold for a moment and then slowly raise your hips back to the starting position by driving through the heel of your right foot. There'll be a tendency to do most of the work by bouncing on the toes of your left foot. Try not to let this happen. You'll end up looking like you're doing the movement correctly, but this compensation will take the focus off the quads.

If you're doing it correctly, you should feel work being done by your right quadriceps and your right glutes and you should get a very deep stretch in your left quadriceps and hip. Work your way up to doing sets of 20 reps on each leg. Once you can do this relatively easily, try doing it carrying light dumbbells in each hand. For the weighted variation, shoot for sets of 15.

Progression: Perform the same movement with the front foot on a balance pad. Definitely make sure you're comfortable with the added balance challenge of this variation before adding any dumbbells to the movement! This progression will add some bonus stability work for the knee and ankle and some extra work for the muscles of the lower leg.

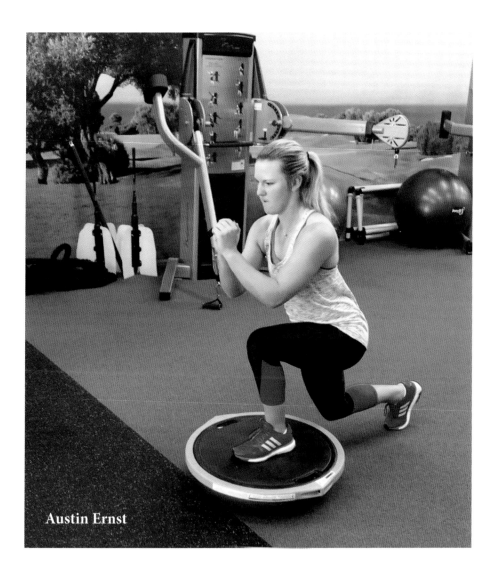

Austin Ernst

Hamstring Curls
HAMSTRING STRENGTH AT THE KNEES

A great exercise for strengthening the hamstrings. If you're working out on a floor, you can use two dish towels for this. If you're working out on carpet, you can use a pair of furniture sliders. They're very inexpensive and can easily be found online or in a hardware store.

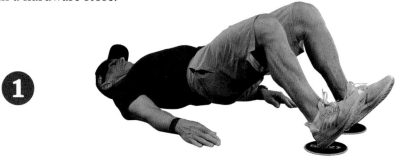

1) Lie on the floor with your knees bent and your feet flat on the ground on either towels or furniture sliders. You should be able to just touch your heels with your fingertips. Without arching your lower back, lift your hips off the ground until there's no bend at the hips and your body is a straight line from your knees to your shoulders. This is the starting position.

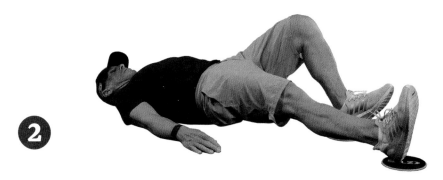

2) Keeping the hips up as much as possible, slide your right foot out until your right leg is almost straight. Try to maintain pressure on the towel or furniture slider as you do this to avoid it slipping away from you. When the right leg is fully extended, begin to pull it back toward you as you let your left leg slide out. The goal is to get a continuous motion going where one leg is sliding out as the other is pulling in. Ideally, when done correctly, you should look like a bug on its back flailing desperately to get back onto its feet. Hey, no one said this was going to be pretty! Try to do sets of 20 alternating curls – 10 with each leg.

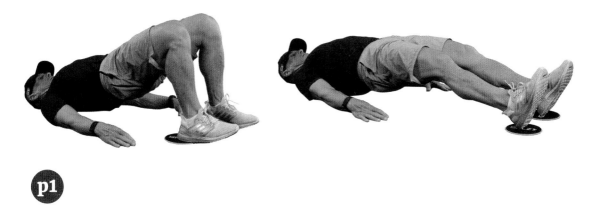

Progression One: To challenge the hamstrings a bit more, try doing the move with both feet moving in and out together. From the same starting position and without dropping your hips or arching your lower back, slowly let your feet slide away from you. When your legs are almost straight, reverse the movement and pull your feet back in toward you. Your hips are going to want to drop when you begin to bring your feet back in. Try not to let that happen. These can be tough. Initially try for sets of 6 to 8 repetitions, but work your way up to sets of 20.

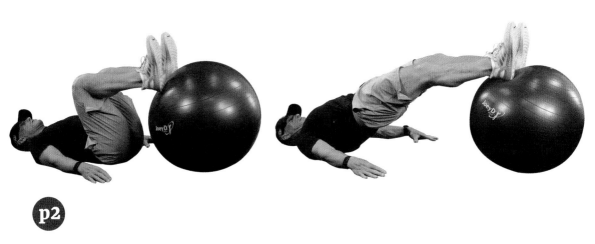

Progression Two: Take Progression One to a new level by doing the movement with your feet on a 55- or 65-centimeter stability ball instead of towels or sliders. Elevating the feet allows for a much greater range of motion for the movement, which will make it a little bit tougher. And placing your feet on something that doesn't want to stay in one place will make it a lot tougher.

"We've done a lot of work to strengthen my hips. Now I have the ability to rotate them through."

LEXI THOMPSON

CHAPTER SIX

The Hips

Our species-specific approach to training focuses on two things: how the human body was originally intended to move and how people actually move today. The goals are to identify the differences between the two and then minimize those differences in order to restore proper movement patterns. And nowhere is it more apparent how human movement has strayed and devolved from its original design than it is when we look at the hips. We've already discussed the ways that our current lifestyles may have affected movement around the ankles and knees, but – at the end of the day – we all know how to use our ankles and knees and we still use them every day.

The hips are another story. Because we sit most of the day and because once we become adults, we rarely have to run very fast on a regular basis, jump really high, or throw things very far, our ability to use and get the most out of our hips has greatly diminished.

While this is sad enough news from a physiological or anthropological standpoint, it's even sadder news if you're a golfer. The ability to properly function around the hips will be the main indicator of how well you'll be able to swing the golf club. Without the ability to control and take advantage of movement at the hips, you might as well ignore the previous two chapters and you might as well start playing golf while sitting in a chair.

When we talk about the hips' role in the golf swing, we're talking about all the possible movements that can occur at the pelvis. And there's lots of them.

Unlike the ankle and the knee where you have one joint around which movement occurs, when we talk about the hips, we're actually talking about three very distinct, but very linked, joints. On the lower half of the pelvis, you have two omnidirectional ball-and-socket joints where the left and right femurs – the large bone of the thigh – attach to the pelvis. At the top of the pelvis, you have the connection to the base of the spine.

You can go online and read all sorts of things about what the most complex joint in the human body is. Some might say it's the shoulder because of the huge range of motion that the arm has. Others might say it's the wrist because of all the very slight and delicate motions that it allows the hand to be able to do.

For our purposes, though, we're going with the hips. Like the shoulders, the ball-and-socket joints where the thigh bone connects to the pelvis allow for all sorts of movement. You can move your leg forward slightly like you do when you walk, or you can bring your knee way up in front of you. You also have a great range of degrees in which you can move your leg in back of you. You can move your leg out to the side and also bring it across your body like you do when you cross your legs.

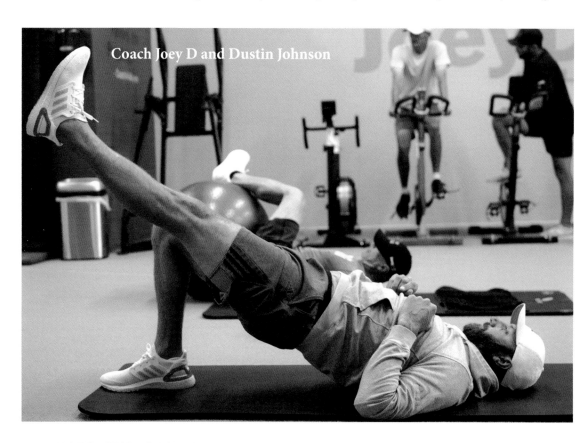
Coach Joey D and Dustin Johnson

The Anatomy of the Hips

A DETAIL OF THE PELVIS AND SURROUNDING AREA

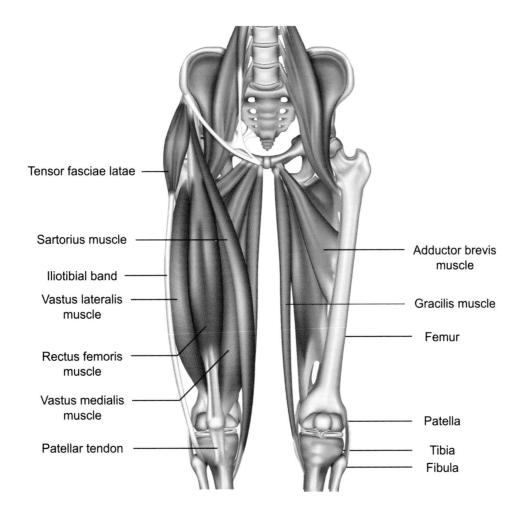

Tensor fasciae latae

Sartorius muscle

Iliotibial band

Vastus lateralis
muscle

Rectus femoris
muscle

Vastus medialis
muscle

Patellar tendon

Adductor brevis
muscle

Gracilis muscle

Femur

Patella

Tibia

Fibula

There's also a lot of rotation that occurs at these ball-and-socket joints. Think about the pivoting that occurs at your foot when you step on a bug or finish your golf swing.

The shoulders can – and very often do – operate independently of each other. You can be doing all sort of things with your left arm, while your right arm does nothing. It's a very rare movement at one hip that doesn't affect the other hip. Very little movement at the hip is done in isolation. When we walk, stepping forward with one leg forces subtle movements to occur at the other leg. (And most movements at the lower part of the pelvis create movement of the spine at the top of the pelvis.) And that's just walking. Think about how synced the two legs have to be when we run, jump, or hit a golf ball. Finally, since most movements at the hip occur while we're standing, this forces movement at the knees, ankles, and feet. If those movements at the knees, ankles, and feet didn't happen, we'd constantly be in an off-balanced state, and we'd probably be falling down a lot more often.

To be able to create and control all this omnidirectional movement, you need a lot of different and specialized muscles. To move the leg forward, you have hip flexors on both the left and right side. (They're also responsible for tilting the pelvis forward as if you were trying to aim your belt buckle at the floor.) To move the leg backward you have the primary hip extensors of the body, your glutes. (The glutes are also responsible for tilting the hips back as if you were trying to get your belt buckle to point to the sky.) Abductor muscles on the outer sides of the hips move the legs outward and away from the body, and adductor muscles on the inside of the thigh pull the leg back toward the midline of your body. There are also numerous smaller muscles that are responsible for internal and external rotation of the leg bone.

You now probably know more than you ever expected to know about the hips, but we're guessing you didn't buy this book solely to bulk up on anatomical trivia. The good news is that now that you understand how the hips move – or at least are supposed to move – it's time to learn how proper function will elevate your game, how dysfunction will harm your game, and what you can do about it.

With all of the potential movement at the hips and so many muscles and muscle groups that have to perform well together, it's not a big surprise that there's a lot of room for dysfunction at the hips. And nothing will expose them more – or as quickly – as the game of golf.

A big problem that we see a lot is a stability issue where a player is unable to control side-to-side movement of the hips. As they go into their backswing, the momentum of the takeaway causes the hips to sway a few inches away from their target and toward the back foot. It's the body's way of trying to stay in balance. The good news is that you won't fall over. The bad news is that you've just taken yourself out of the proper swing plane. You're now behind the ball and have to hope that the forward momentum of your downswing will put your hips in EXACTLY the right spot at impact. That's a lot to expect on a regular basis. Odds are when there's a lot of side-to-side sway, there's going to be accuracy issues. Remember, motion at the hips creates motion at the knees and ankles, so if there's extra unnecessary movement at the hips, there's also going to be extra movement in a bunch of other places. That's a lot of extra moving parts to add to an already complex movement! If you're in complete control of the side-to-side movement of the hips, you can remove a lot of chaos from your swing.

"When I work with my swing coach now on making adjustments, it's so much easier now. I feel like I can control my body much better." – **Azahara Muñoz**

Another big concern has more to do with mobility – actually, lack of mobility – and how it affects golf posture. If your hips naturally tilt forward, this can force an unnatural overarching of the lower back that's going to restrict proper rotation. So, how do you know if your hips are tilted forward? A good test is to see where your belt buckle is facing. If it's facing downward or toward the floor instead of straight ahead, your hips are tilted forward. This anterior shift is another result of us sitting too much. And if you're a few pounds overweight and you're carrying that extra weight in your stomach, that's another factor that can lead to a forward tilting pelvis.

But it's not much better if your hips tilt backward. Is your belt buckle facing upward instead of straight ahead? If so, your lower back is now rounded. And the only way you're going to get into anything close to golf posture is by rounding your upper back at the top of the spine. This rounded, C-shaped back almost guarantees that you won't be able to rotate properly through your swing. So, whether your hips are tilted too far forward or too far backward, either dysfunction is going to negatively affect accuracy and consistency in your game.

The biggest problem, though, is when a player is unable to get any movement at the hips. Unlike the previous two dysfunctions that will simply make your time out on the course less fun, not being able to rotate at the hips has a really good chance of making your time off the course a lot less fun, as well.

I'm sure you've seen very arms-y players. Some might even be decent golfers despite having a dysfunctional – and pretty ugly – swing. If you're an arms-y player and you can shoot a decent round, consider yourself lucky (although you're not playing anywhere near your potential). If you're an arms-y player and you haven't injured your lower back, consider yourself incredibly lucky.

When the swing is done almost entirely with the upper body, a few things happen. First of all, you're never going to get the same clubhead speed as you would if you were rotating properly through the hips. You don't need to be a physicist to know that a slower clubhead at impact is going to result in less ball speed and less distance. That's the bad news on the golf course. More importantly, repeatedly trying to launch bombs by rotating only at the spine – and not at the hips – is almost certain to injure your lower back. The lower portion of the spine – the lumbar spine – isn't designed to be as mobile or to be able to rotate as much as the mid-spine, but that doesn't stop a lot of golfers from trying to make it rotate more than it should.

> *"At some point in the season, I would always struggle with lower back pain. Pretty much since working with Kolby, other than getting off a plane after 15 hours, I've had no back pain at all. Injury-wise, I've never felt better. I think his eye for how the body moves and how golfers should move and what my limitations are is incredible. He has the best eye for that I've ever seen."*
> – **Austin Ernst**

Think about how much your shoulders turn from address through your backswing and then from your downswing through impact and follow-through. That's a lot of rotation. To make sure that this is done in a safe way, ideally, your hips rotate about 45 degrees away from your target during your backswing. This will generally allow you to get about 90 degrees of rotation around the spine. Through impact and into your follow-through, the hips rotate about 135 degrees toward your target. Meanwhile, your thoracic spine will rotate approximately 180 degrees from the top of your backswing through impact and into your follow-through.

Now imagine trying to get that much rotation without the hips helping out. What you get is a prescription for back pain. Despite the fact that their hips aren't turning, players still feel like they have to look like the picture of the golfer in the magazine or the pro playing on TV – a giant takeaway and a wrap-the-club-around-your-neck follow-through. It ends up being an incredible amount of explosive rotation around body parts that just weren't meant to rotate this much or this dynamically all by themselves.

The good news is that if you've read the previous couple of chapters, you'll know that if there's correct movement at the ankles and knees, there's a better chance that there'll be proper movement at the hips. Increasing the mobility, stability, and strength around the hips is an invaluable way to not only improve your game, but also to improve your quality of life both on and off the course.

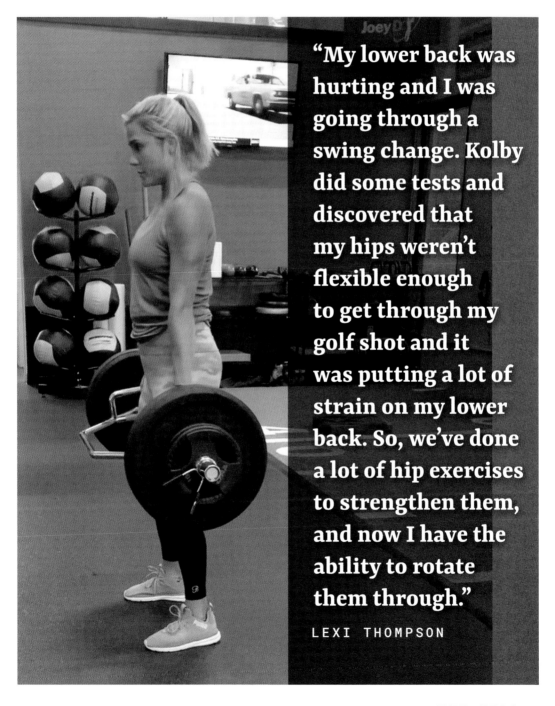

"My lower back was hurting and I was going through a swing change. Kolby did some tests and discovered that my hips weren't flexible enough to get through my golf shot and it was putting a lot of strain on my lower back. So, we've done a lot of hip exercises to strengthen them, and now I have the ability to rotate them through."

LEXI THOMPSON

Hip Tilt with Stability Ball

HIP MOBILITY

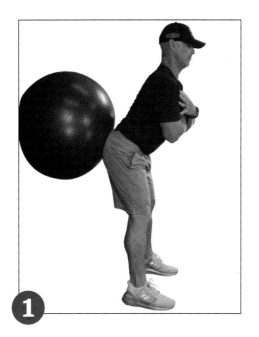 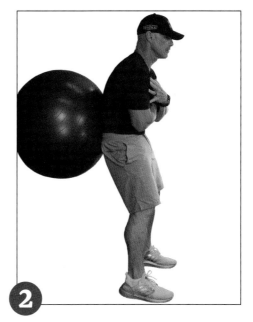

To get a feel for the muscles that control the forward and backward tilting of your pelvis – and to help you correct postural issues that will negatively affect your game – place a 55- or 65-centimeter stability ball against a wall and press your lower back against it. Without letting the ball fall to the ground, assume an address position with good posture and spine angle. This is the starting position.

1) Slowly and with good control, tilt your hips forward as if you were trying to point your belt buckle toward the floor. Try to avoid any other movement. When you do this, you should feel the ball sliding slightly up your back. Hold this for a three-count.

2) Reverse the move and tilt your hips as far back as possible, as if you were trying to point your belt buckle toward the ceiling. You might feel tension in your glutes when you do this – and that's a good thing! Again, watch for any other body parts like your knees or your back trying to help out. You should feel the ball sliding down your back when you do this. Hold this position for a three-count and then tilt your hips slightly forward until you are back to the starting position to complete the rep.

Feeling the movement of the ball is a great way to tell that you're doing the move correctly. And by staying in golf posture, it will help remove a lot of the potential compensations that may want to happen. Over time, you'll find that you're able to go deeper into each direction, which is proof of not only a greater and increased range of motion, but also of your ability to control the movement of your hips, which is an invaluable skill on the golf course. Shoot for 10 repetitions.

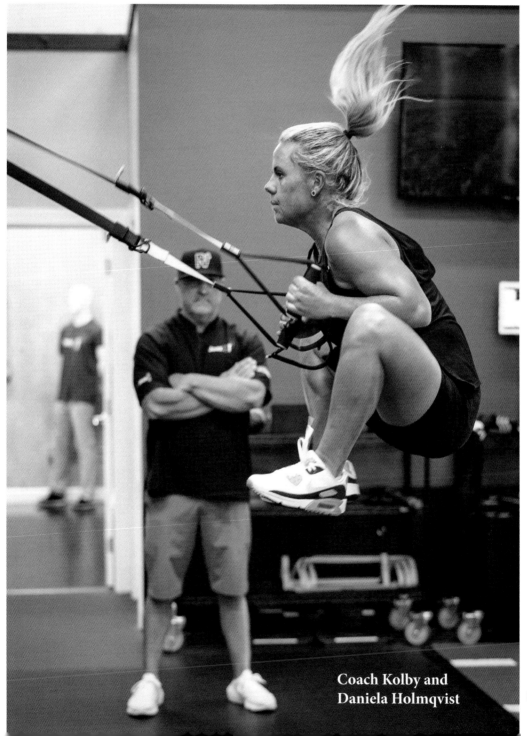

Coach Kolby and
Daniela Holmqvist

Standing Hip Opener
HIP MOBILITY

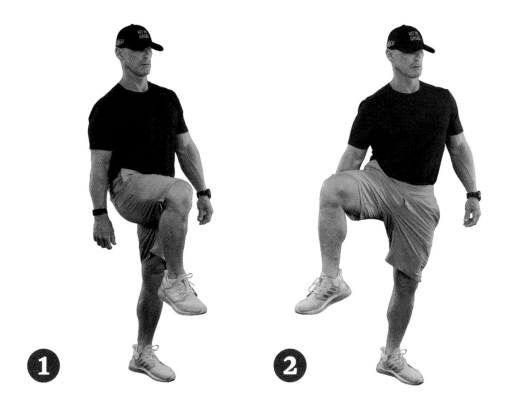

1) To get your hips used to internal and external rotation, stand with your feet shoulder-width apart. Toes should be facing forward. This is the starting position. Raise your right leg so that your thigh is at waist height and parallel to the floor. Establish balance in this position.

2) Slowly rotate your right leg outward until your knee is aimed directly to your right. Try to do this without turning your entire body. In other words, while your knee may be facing to the right, your hips, chest, and shoulders are still squared forward. Hold for a three-count and then return to the starting position. You'll not only feel this in the hips, but also in your core. These are the muscles that are working to prevent your upper body from rotating toward the moving leg. Do 10 hip openers on each side.

Lateral Movement with Looped Band

HIP STABILITY

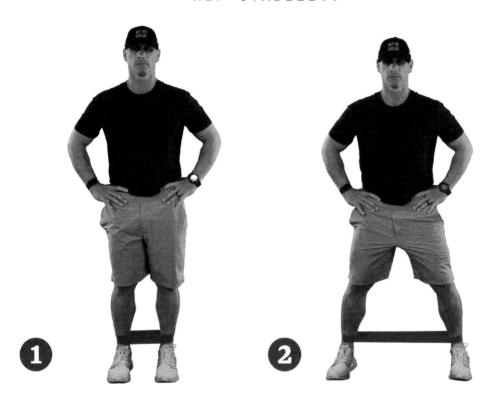

Even if you go to the gym on a regular basis, there's still a good chance that you're not targeting the muscles on the outsides of the hips. These are the muscles that are going to help you control side-to-side movement of the hips during your swing.

1) Put a looped resistance band around your ankles and stand with your feet about six inches apart. Even with this narrow stance, there should be a tiny bit of tension in the band. This is the starting position.

2) Keeping your toes pointed forward, step sideways with your right leg into a slightly wider than shoulder-width stance. You should quickly feel some awareness at the sides of your hips. It's key that the toes face forward throughout the movement. There's going to be a tendency to turn your right foot out as you step. If this happens, then it becomes your hip flexors that are doing the work. We don't want them doing the work here. By keeping the toes forward, it guarantees that your hip abductors on the outside part of the hip are being engaged. Hold this stance for a beat and then step your left foot toward your right foot until you're back in the starting position. Take five steps to the right and then five steps to the left to complete each set.

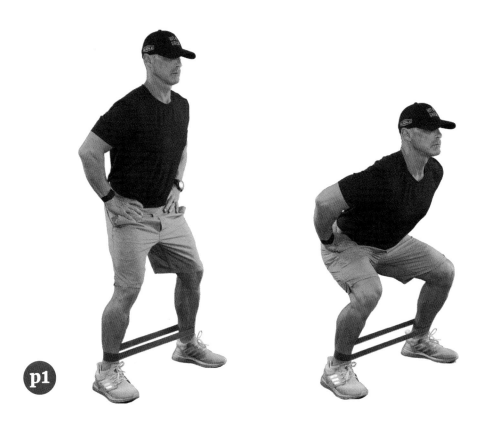

Progression One: From the same starting position, step into a slightly wider than shoulder-width stance with your right foot and instead of simply holding the position, throw your hips back and – keeping your knees directly over your heels – drop into a squat position. Keeping your knees directly over your heels will not only keep your knees healthy, it will also force your quads and glutes to work harder. You might also feel your knees caving in toward each other. By preventing this from happening and keeping your knees wide apart, you're getting your hip abductors on the outside of the hip to work harder. Hold the squat position for a moment and slowly come out of the squat and back into the slightly wider than shoulder-width stance. Step your left foot toward your right foot to return to the starting position. Adding a squat to the movement will add extra work for the muscles on the sides of the hips as well as a good amount of glute work. Try for sets of five step-and-squats to each side.

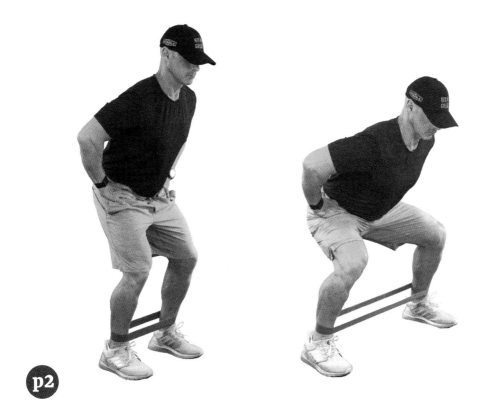

Progression Two: Similar to the movement on the previous page, but instead of breaking the move into four parts, try to break it into only two parts. From the same starting position, step into a slightly wider than shoulder-width stance at the same time that you're lowering your hips into a squat. Hold the squat for a moment and then simultaneously come out of the squat and step your left foot toward your right until you're back to the starting position. There's a lot going on with this progression, so make sure you've mastered Progression One before moving on to this one. As previously, shoot for sets of five side-stepping squats to both the right and the left.

Hip Bridges

GLUTE STRENGTH AT THE HIPS

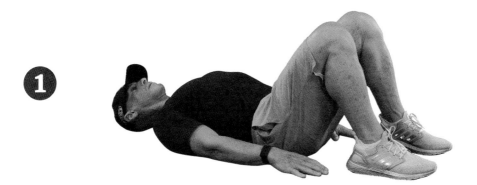

1) Lie on your back with your knees bent and your feet flat on the ground. If you reach down, you should just be able to touch your heels.

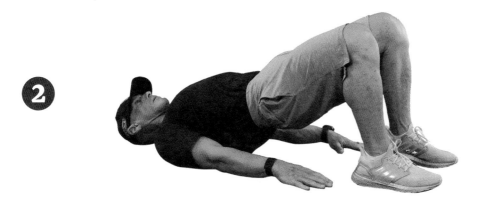

2) Without arching your lower back, slowly lift your hips off the ground. See if you're able to lift them so that your body forms a straight line from your knees to your shoulders. You might feel a nice stretch across the tops of your hips and quadriceps here. Hold this for a second and then return to the starting position. As you get stronger, instead of returning to the completely relaxed starting position, lower yourself until your back is an inch from the ground before beginning the next hip raise. Initially, shoot for sets of 10, but don't be afraid to challenge yourself with as many as 25 reps as long as you can keep proper form without any lower back arching.

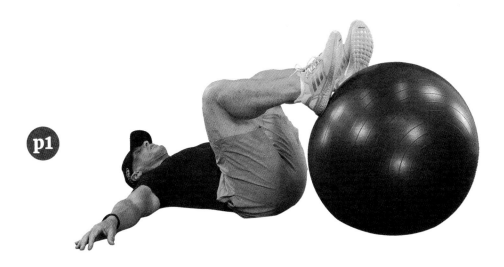

Progression One: Perform the same movement with your feet flat on top of a 55- or 65-centimeter stability ball about hip-width apart. (Depending on the size of the ball, you may not be able to completely flatten your foot on top of the ball in the setup position.)

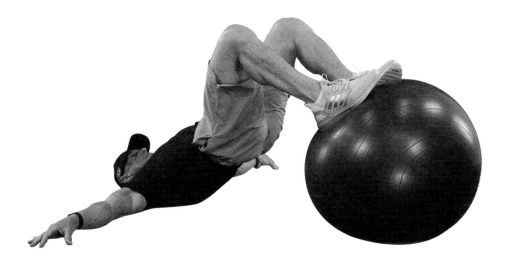

You'll want to extend your arms out to the sides with palms down to help with balance. You will feel this almost immediately in your hamstrings and calves. Try not to let your knees cave in toward each other or bow out. Ideally, the distance between your knees should be the same as the distance between your feet. Shoot for 10 to 15 reps.

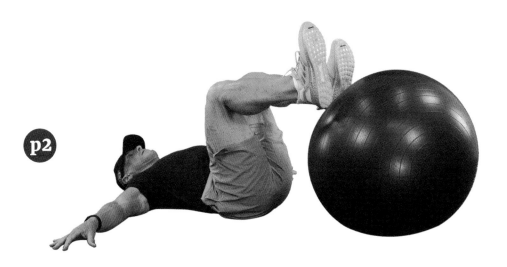

Progression Two: Set up as in the first progression, but with your feet very close to each other on the ball.

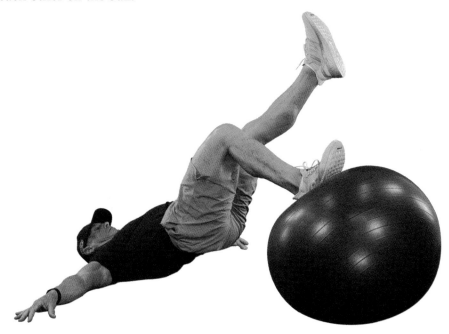

Lift your hips off the floor as before, but this time slowly straighten your left leg toward the ceiling. To keep your lower back in proper position, keep your left leg slightly bent with your knee directly above your navel. Keeping the left leg raised and very quiet, slowly lower your body until your back is an inch off the ground and then return to the raised hip position. You will feel this very profoundly in your right hamstring and calf and your balance will definitely be challenged. These will be tough, but try for 8 to 10 reps.

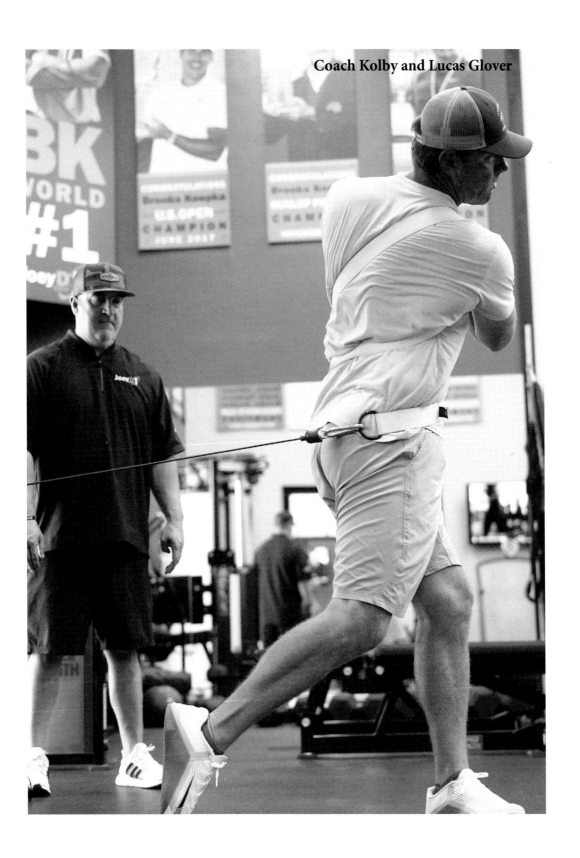

Coach Kolby and Lucas Glover

"It's just become a part of my life. I really do love working out and I enjoy the grind."

JUSTIN THOMAS

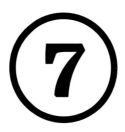

CHAPTER SEVEN

The Spine

Most of the bony structures in the body are pretty simple and their roles are fairly obvious. The job of the femur – the thigh bone – is to connect the bones of the lower leg to the pelvis. The job of the humerus – the bone of the upper arm – is to connect the bones of the forearm to the bones that make up the shoulder complex. The job of the teeth is to chew. The spine, though, is a whole lot more interesting. It's the body's skeletal multitasker. And compared to the other bony structures that we'll cover, the spine is a lot more complex and delicate and is a lot more vital and important for maintaining a healthy and happy lifestyle.

The spine is a chain of 33 small, somewhat donut-shaped, vertically stacked bones. One of its jobs is to keep the body upright and connect the bones of the lower body to those of the upper body. It's also the attachment point of the ribs, whose job it is to protect the heart and lungs. And as if that wasn't already enough, it also has the monumental responsibility of housing and protecting the spinal cord, which snakes vertically through the "donut holes" of the spine.

It's divided up into five sections. The uppermost seven vertebrae make up the cervical spine. It's the most flexible region of the spine and we'll be getting more into the cervical spine when we talk about the neck.

Just below the cervical spine are the 12 vertebrae that make up the thoracic spine. Often referred to as the mid-spine, this is where the majority of spinal rotation occurs. Below the thoracic spine are the five larger vertebrae that make up the lumbar spine. If you read the previous chapter, we talked about the lumbar spine's relationship with the pelvis. Below the lumbar spine are five fused-together vertebrae that make up the sacral spine, which is where the actual connection to the pelvis occurs. Finally, there are the four fused vertebrae that make up the tailbone. All told, when you take out the two fused sections, you end up with a structure that's essentially a string of about two dozen individual joints – each vertebra's functionality or dysfunctionality affecting the vertebrae above it and the vertebrae below it.

The individual vertebrae are numbered by the particular area of the spine they're in. If you've ever been told by a doctor that you have issues with L3 or L4, they would be referring to the third and fourth vertebrae in the lumbar spine or lower back. If the doctor knew golf, he'd be able to guess that you might be a very arms-y player.

Between each of the vertebrae from the second cervical vertebrae down to the bottom of the lumbar spine are disks that cushion the movement of the bones that make up the spine and prevent bone on bone contact.

For a multitude of reasons, we want to keep your spine happy. Slight dysfunction at the spine can result in muscular issues that may be long-lasting and nagging. More intense dysfunction can result in damage to the disks that serve as cushioning

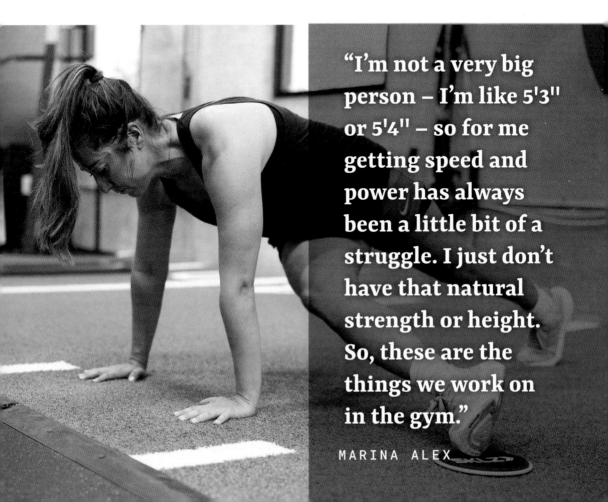

"I'm not a very big person – I'm like 5'3" or 5'4" – so for me getting speed and power has always been a little bit of a struggle. I just don't have that natural strength or height. So, these are the things we work on in the gym."

MARINA ALEX

The Anatomy of the Spine

A DETAIL OF THE SPINAL AREAS

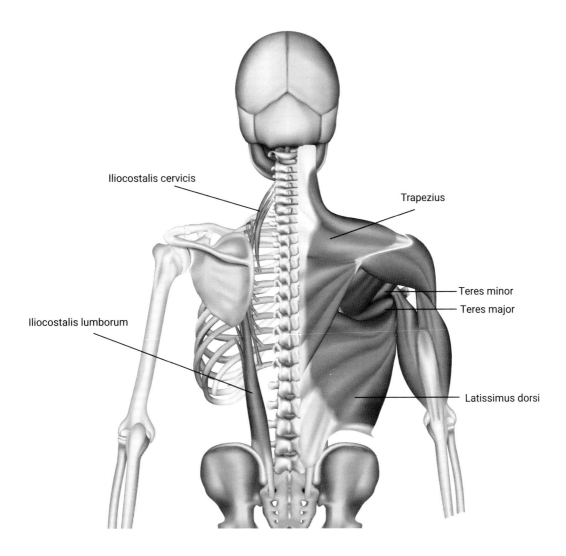

Iliocostalis cervicis

Trapezius

Teres minor

Teres major

Iliocostalis lumborum

Latissimus dorsi

between the vertebrae. A herniated disk can mean sharp chronic pain or numbness and a lifetime of over-the-counter and prescription medicines. Serious trauma may result in damage to the spinal cord, which could result in partial or full paralysis.

We mentioned some of the ways the lower spine can be affected by improper hip movement in the previous chapter. This chapter will focus primarily on the thoracic or mid-spine. And, happily, the odds of you doing any real damage to your mid-spine out on the golf course are relatively slim. That doesn't mean that you don't

Nervous Energy

The spinal cord, along with the brain, make up the central nervous system. If you want to think of the brain as the main headquarters where all the input from your senses is analyzed and interpreted and where all of the information and instructions heading to the muscles and organs of the body originates, then you can think of the spinal cord as the main highway leading in and out of this headquarters.

The spinal cord, itself, is housed and protected by the spine. It originates in the brain and travels down through the spine and ends in the lumbar vertebrae. Openings in the vertebrae allow the fibers of the central nervous system to connect to nerve fibers of the peripheral nervous system – the pathway of nerves that connect to the muscles, internal organs, and sensory organs of the body.

Every bodily movement, regardless how big or small, is regulated and controlled by the nervous system. A lot of the work is done without us really thinking about it. The body is essentially on "cruise control" when it comes to breathing, digestion, and the beating of your heart. Some of the work is done with a minimum of awareness – your face scrunches up when you smell something bad, you mindlessly scratch an itch, etc. And some is done with full awareness – your foot slowly stepping on the gas pedal and your hands and arms turning the steering wheel only after your brain has decided it's safe to take a left-hand turn based on information taken in through the eyes and ears.

To be able to reach every part of the body, you need to have a pretty complex network of nerves. Unlike our muscles and bones, though, our nerves toil away in relative anonymity. Very few people have ever said, "Wow. My oculomotor nerve is firing on all cylinders today!" after being able to read some extremely fine print. In fact, of the hundreds of nerves in the body, maybe the only nerve most people have ever heard of is the sciatic nerve, mainly because when it's impinged upon, it sends pain radiating down the leg. If you've been paying attention, this would be what we would consider a dysfunction, because – ideally – you're not supposed to have pain radiating down your leg. In the case of the sciatic nerve, the dysfunction occurs with its relationship with the piriformis muscle in the hip.

If you remember from Chapter 3, our goal isn't just to develop and strengthen the body in a logical and balanced way, but also to challenge the nervous system. By continually getting the body to adapt to new neuromuscular challenges, we can make huge improvements in balance, coordination, body awareness, and other intangibles that will make you more effective out on the course.

have to pay attention to what your spine is doing when you're lining up your tee shot; it just means that of all the ways that you can hurt yourself with a golf club in your hands, an injury to your thoracic spine isn't high up on the list. Your ability to move and control movement at the spine, though, will directly affect whether your ball finds the fairway or not.

"Coming back from my accident, I couldn't even address the ball with my side being so swollen from the broken ribs. We did a lot of core and back things to get everything working together. And, finally, I was able to get my full turn back. I still have good days and bad days, but overall, I feel 100 percent and just as good as I did before." – Bud Cauley

Most of the strength and stability issues around the spine have to do with posture. Maintaining good golf posture from address through takeaway and from your downswing to your follow-through is the key to accuracy. Anything that takes you out of proper posture is going to affect your swing plane, and that's going to determine where your ball is going to end up.

Most people that have questionable posture aren't even aware of it. And if you don't know that your posture is less than spectacular in an upright position, there's even less of a chance that you're going to realize that your posture is suspect in a more contrived position – like it is during the golf swing.

To begin to remedy this, we do things that create awareness of the muscles of the back. Once again due to our lifestyles, a lot of people have no connection to their back and their posture. We hunch over keyboards all day and we spend our free time with our chins buried in our chests looking at our phones. It's not a major surprise that a lot of us have weakness around the spine and, as a result, postural issues.

But even people who do go to the gym may inadvertently be doing things that increase – and not decrease – postural issues. A lot of people in the gym only work on the things they can see in the mirror – the chest, the shoulders, the biceps, the abs. The result is that they essentially exercise their way out of shape. Focusing on just the front of the body creates imbalance, and imbalance leads to dysfunction. Overly tight muscles in the chest and abs coupled with a lifestyle that's loaded with a lot of computer time and phone gazing is a recipe for a forward-rounded posture.

One of the keys to improving the ability to maintain proper posture is developing the muscles in the back of the body. Like most rotational sports, golf is a "posterior chain" sport, which means that success is going to depend on the strength of the muscles in the back of your body. (The ones you can't see in the mirror.) These are the muscles that keep the spine upright and not pitched forward. You've probably heard of the latissimus dorsi – or "lats" – but deeper postural muscles that we also need to focus on strengthening include the rhomboids, which pull the shoulder blades back and lets you squeeze them together, and the trapezius, which is responsible for upward, backward, and downward motion of the shoulder blades.

And the goal for strengthening these muscles is twofold. In addition to simply creating muscular strength, we need to be concentrating on improving muscular endurance, as well. It's great that you're able to have perfect posture on the course for the first nine, but if the muscles responsible for that great posture don't have endurance, your back nine is going to be another story.

With a bent-over or C-shaped spine, the inability to maintain good posture will throw your swing plane into chaos. With a rounded back, you tend to become more

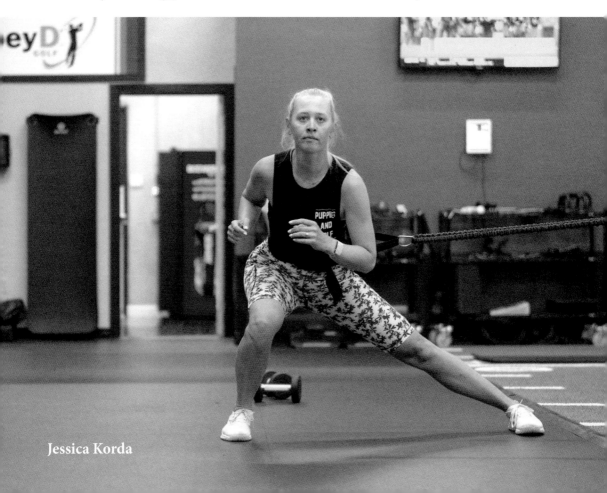

Jessica Korda

upright during your downswing and you decelerate the hips. You're going to hit the ball thin and with less power. The irregular swing plane created by a forward-curved spine will also make it tough to predict where your club face will be at impact, leading to accuracy issues.

"In 2013 in my first year on what's now the Korn Ferry Tour, I led the tour in scoring average and greens-in-regulation. I was top five in birdies, top five in total driving, and top five in another one. And that was all a drastic improvement from the year before. I went from being a below average player to being one of the best on the tour within a year, and all of that was due to Kolby." – John Peterson

Mobility issues arise when we see a player with a limited ability to rotate around their spine. Again, our lifestyles are to blame. We sit all day and when we want to turn around, instead of actually turning around, we just swivel our chairs in whatever direction we want. The result of this sedentary lifestyle is that we lose the ability to rotate around the spine.

Good spinal mobility sets you up for proper rotation in the golf swing. In your backswing, when your hips turn away from your target, it's that spinal mobility that gives you 90 degrees of thoracic rotation into your backswing. If you've ever read or had a coach tell you that they wanted you to get your back to the target, you understand how important it is to improve your ability to rotate around your spine. The farther back you can rotate away from your target, the more clubhead speed you can build.

To take maximum advantage of this potential for power, velocity, and speed, you need the ability to create a sufficient amount of rotation, giving you ample time for a dynamic follow-through. If your body doesn't allow you to rotate through the end of your swing, you'll end up decelerating early. And this means sacrificing speed and power.

Think about it this way. Have you ever seen an Olympic 100-meter race? After they cross the finish line, runners decelerate slowly and end up running about 200 meters in total. But what would it look like if there was a stone wall 10 meters past the finish line? Runners would start decelerating at about the 60-meter mark out of self-preservation. (Or, more likely, they would just find a safer sport.) Golfers need time to decelerate their swing. If you don't have the time to do it comfortably after impact, then you're going to be doing it before impact, which – obviously – isn't an optimal situation.

Of course, not everyone is going to get exactly these numbers – and some might get even more rotation due to being hypermobile – but the goal is to get as close as possible. But remember, all this rotation has to take place in the proper places in the body – the hips, lower spine, and mid-spine.

If a player can't get that much rotation in the mid-back, a couple of things might happen. They may try to wrench some more turn out of their lower spine, which is one of the dysfunctions we talked about in the previous chapter, or they may try to make up for the lack of movement with exaggerated arm movement. The arms-ier the swing becomes, the less powerful it becomes. Fortunately, creating mobility and movement around the mid-spine isn't an impossible thing to do. It's not a quick fix, though. Unless it was due to an accident, trauma, or surgery, people don't tend to lose the ability to rotate overnight. So, it shouldn't be assumed you'll be able to regain that ability to rotate overnight.

Intelligently working to increase range of motion around the mid-spine is definitely worth the investment. Your game will improve and you'll have a lot more fun and a lot less pain out on the course. And, off the course, you'll find that life just becomes a lot easier when you have that added mobility at the spine.

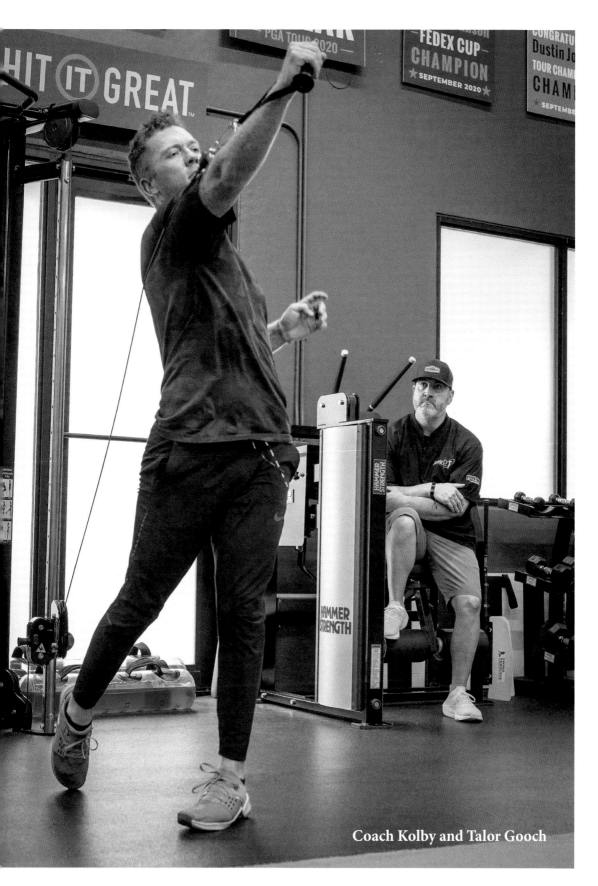

Coach Kolby and Talor Gooch

Cat/Cow Stretch

SPINAL MOBILITY

A great way to help undo the effects of our seated sedentary lifestyle and a great way to increase spinal flexion and extension – or the forward and backward bending of the spine.

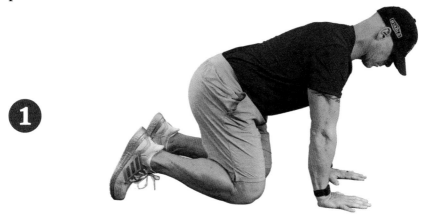

1) Get onto all fours. Your hands should be directly under your shoulders and your knees should be directly under your hips.

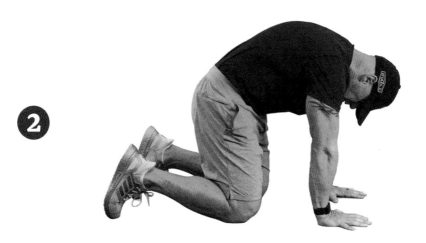

2) Slowly round your back as far as you can do comfortably. Imagine trying to touch the middle of your back to the ceiling. This will involve more than just the muscles alongside the spine, you'll feel a stretch into your hips and shoulders, as well. This is the "cat" portion of the move.

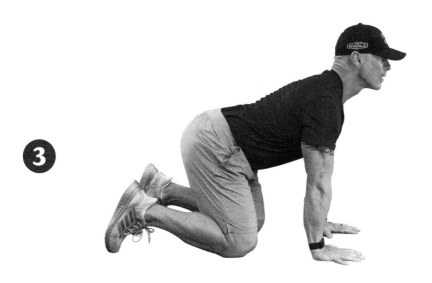

3) Now, slowly reverse the movement and arch your back as if you were trying to drop your stomach to the floor. This is the "cow" portion. You may feel more restriction in this part of the exercise – especially in the lower back. Hold this position for a moment and then transfer back to the "cat" phase by rounding your back again. Continue until you've done 10 "cats" and 10 "cows." Don't be surprised if you're able to go deeper into each move as your body loosens. We guarantee you will feel better after doing this than you did before you started. It's that good of a movement.

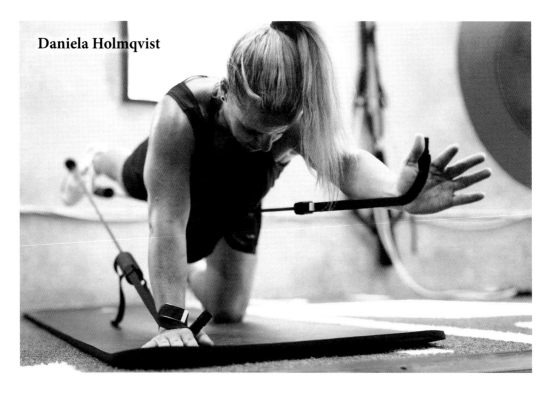

Daniela Holmqvist

Follow-Through with Bands

SPINAL MOBILITY

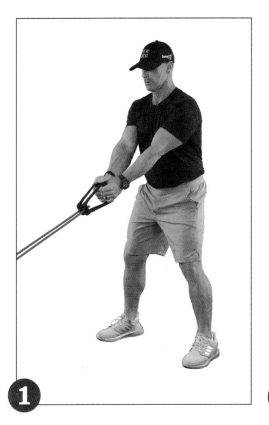

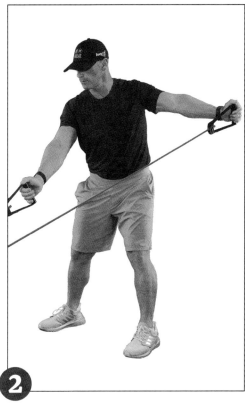

1) To increase rotational mobility of the spine, attach a double-handled V-shaped resistance band to a knee-high anchor point. Stand facing the anchor point in address position with a handle in each hand with your palms facing in and toward each other. Your arms should be extended in front of you and angled toward the anchor point as if they were extensions of the bands. There should be slight tension in the bands. This is the starting position.

2) Keeping your left arm straight, dynamically rotate your arm and upper body to the left. Since you're trying to simulate a follow-through-like movement, pivot on

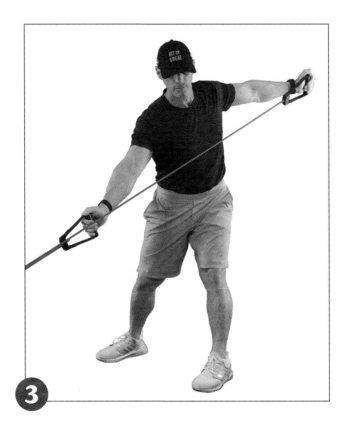

the ball of the right foot to allow the hips to aid in rotation. Try to keep your right arm still and angled at the anchor point.

3) Since we want to involve the entire spine, rotate your head to the left, as well, as if you were trying to see your ball landing far down the fairway. You should get a deep stretch across the chest and into the shoulders. Reverse the motion and return to the starting position in a controlled fashion – don't just let the tension in the band whip you back to the starting position. Now, do the same move to the right as if you were a left-handed player finishing their swing. Do 10 follow-throughs to both sides.

Standing Anti-Rotation with Bands

SPINAL STABILITY

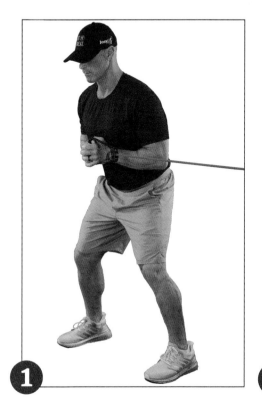 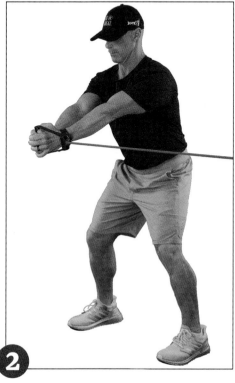

Obviously, one of the jobs of the muscles that act around the spine is to create movement; we've gone into great length to point out the advantages of a mobile spine. Just as important, though, is the ability to stabilize the spine to prevent unwanted movement.

1) Stand holding the handle of a single resistance band in both hands. The anchor point of the band should be at chest height and instead of it being in front of you, it should be directly to your left. Your feet, hips, chest, and shoulders should be squared forward. Hold the handle up against your chest with bent elbows. There should be a decent amount of tension in the band. This is the starting position.

2) Slowly, push your hands out in a straight line from your chest until they're extended directly in front of you. You should feel a good amount of torque pulling you to the left in this arms-extended position. Don't let your arms, chest, hips, knees, or anything else rotate to the left. Hold this position for 10 seconds and then return to the starting position to complete the repetition. You'll feel this in your midsection. Do four holds with the anchor point to your left and then do four holds with the band anchored to your right.

Progression One: Perform the same move as above, but instead of holding the arms-extended position for a ten-count, hold it for a three-count and then return to the starting position to complete the rep. The added movement will add to the challenge of keeping your body from being rotated by the band. In addition to keeping your body quiet, the other major challenge is to move your hands in a perfectly straight line forward in front of you as you extend your arms. The body will try to come up with very creative ways to "cheat" this movement by taking a curving route. This is a tough one when done correctly. If you're finding it very easy to do, double-check to make sure your entire body is squared forward and that your hands are following a straight path away from and back toward your chest. If you're still finding it easy, then you have a really stable spine! Do 10 repetitions with the band anchored to the right and then 10 repetitions with the band anchored to the left.

Progression Two: Perform the same movements as in the above progression, but instead of being in an upright standing position, do the move in golf posture. You'll feel it in your legs, hips, core, and back. This is a great way to create the feeling of full-body stabilization in your address position. Again, 10 reps with a right-side anchored band and 10 reps with a left-side anchored band to complete the set.

Standing Row
with Bands

LATISSIMUS DORSI & RHOMBOID STRENGTH AT THE SPINE

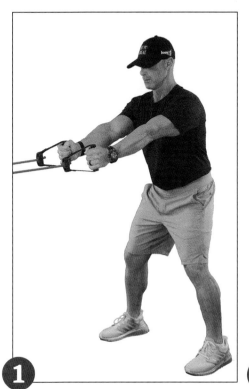
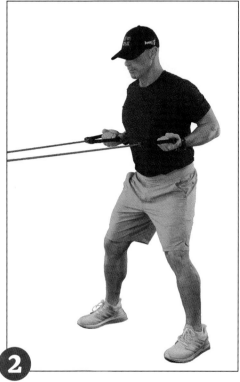

To build both the larger and smaller postural muscles in the back, attach a double-handled V-shaped resistance band to a waist-high anchor point. You can go with a higher resistance band for this one.

1) Face the anchor point with a handle in each hand. Bend your knees slightly and assume an athletic stance – feet a bit wider than shoulder-width apart, hips back, upper body slightly leaning forward with a strong and straight spine. There should be some tension in the bands. This is the starting point.

2) Dynamically pull the bands back by drawing your elbows and shoulder blades back, turning your palms up as you pull. Try not to lose the slight forward lean of your upper body. Your arms should be the only things moving. Hold this pull position for a three-count being aware of keeping your shoulder blades squeezed together. Very slowly, reverse the initial pulling motion to return to the starting position. Let this last part of the move take several seconds.

This move involves the three ways that a muscle can be challenged. The initial quick pull is a concentric contraction and has the muscles in your back (as well as your biceps) shortening against resistance in a very explosive way. The hold with your shoulder blades squeezed together is an isometric contraction, where the muscles have to hold a shortened position against resistance. The slow-motion finish to the move is an example of an eccentric contraction, where the muscles slowly lengthen against resistance. And having your palms facing up the entire time keeps the chest a little more open. There's a lot of good in this exercise. Shoot for 10 rows per set.

Progression: Perform the same movement as above, but in golf posture with the anchor point set below knee-level. The slightly deeper lean that this will force your upper body into will make this version a little more challenging on the muscles of the back. But it's a great way to strengthen the muscles that you'll need to maintain proper posture from the first tee to the last.

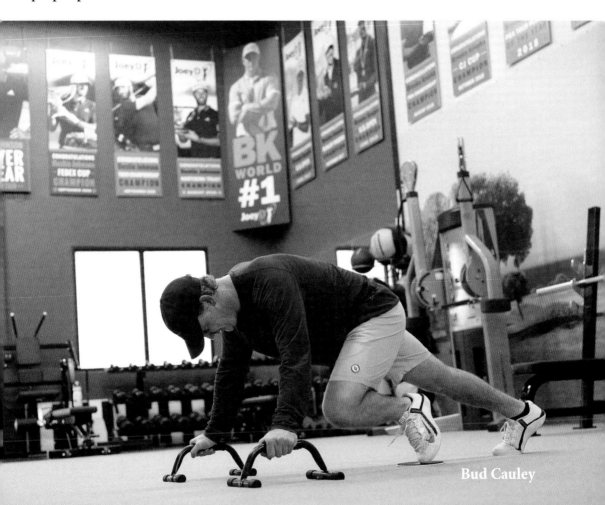

Bud Cauley

Single Arm Row on One Foot

LATISSIMUS DORSI STRENGTH AT THE SPINE

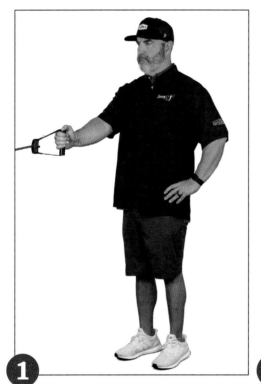 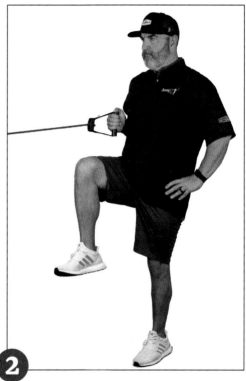

1) To strengthen the postural muscles of the back while also working on lower body strength and balance, attach a resistance band to a chest-high anchor point. Face the anchor point in a very tall, upright stance with the band in your right hand with your palm facing toward the left. There should be slight tension in the band. Raise your right leg so that your right thigh is waist-height and parallel to the floor. This is the starting position.

2) Slowly pull the band back by drawing your elbow and shoulder blade back. Hold this position for a beat and then reverse the movement to return to the starting position to complete the repetition. Try to remain tall and minimize any movement other than your right arm. Your right hip will want to rotate forward or backward. Use the strength in your hips to prevent this. You might also feel this in your left foot as it's working hard to keep you from falling over. Do 10 reps of one-legged rows on each side.

Progression: If you thought that maintaining your balance was difficult in the previous movement, try doing it standing on the leg on the same side of the hand that's pulling. Standing on the right leg while doing the row with the right arm is an adventure in balance. The good news is that if you can master this movement, you'll not only be strengthening the postural muscles around the spine, you'll also be one step closer to having the balancing skills of a mountain goat. As above, shoot for 10 reps on each side.

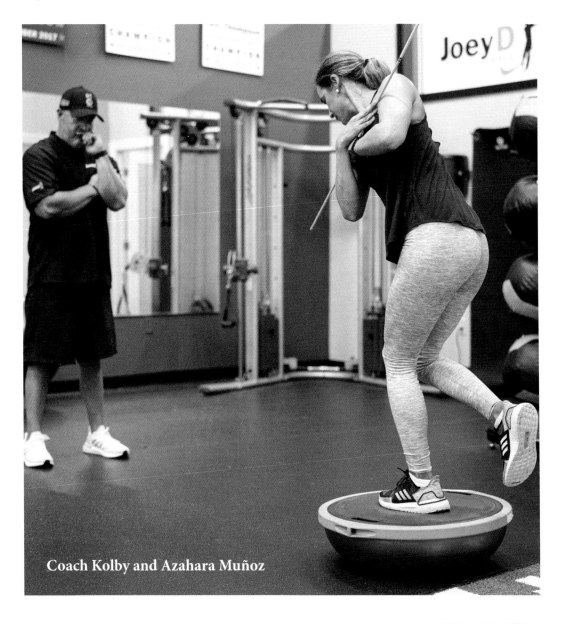

Coach Kolby and Azahara Muñoz

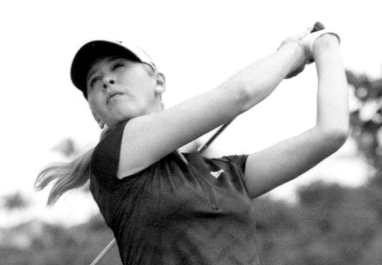

"I underwent jaw surgery right after the 2017 season. Kolby's goal was to get me training and competing within three months. I actually ended up winning my first tournament back and I've been pretty consistent since."

JESSICA KORDA

Jenna Saint Martin

CHAPTER EIGHT

The Neck & Head

Usually, when people talk about the head's role in the golf game, it's in reference to the psychological side of the game. We've all heard Arnold Palmer's famous quote: "Golf is a game of inches. The most important are the six inches between your ears." The head can be the site of some great internal battles – confidence versus self-doubt, courage versus fear. But we're going to look at the head in a far less romantic way. We're looking at the head as the 10- to 12-pound orb perched atop your spine. And your ability to control your head is going to determine just how well you swing a golf club.

When we look at the head and neck, we get some very distinct and clear-cut issues that involve stability, mobility, and strength. The musculature around the head and neck has to be strong enough to stabilize the head and prevent unwanted movement, but also mobile enough to allow required movement. Weakness or tightness will negatively affect your game.

The neck is the uppermost portion of the spine – the cervical spine. It's the most mobile section of the spine and made up of seven vertebrae. (And, interestingly, almost all mammals have seven cervical vertebrae. This includes the giraffe, whose neck averages six feet in length and can weigh upward of 600 pounds.) The extra mobility allowed by these vertebrae allow us to get a lot of movement at the head. We can tilt our heads forward and back as if we're nodding yes. We can rotate our heads from side to side as if we're shaking our heads no. We can tilt our head to the side so that our ear touches our shoulder as if we were trying to understand and appreciate a piece of abstract art. And we can also jut our head forward and retract it backward as if we were pretending to be a pigeon.

All this movement requires some very specialized hardware. The uppermost cervical vertebra (C1) is called the "atlas" because like the Greek hero who was forced to hold up the weight of the world, this topmost vertebra has to support the weight of the head. It works in conjunction with the second cervical vertebra (C2), called the "axis," to form the atlanto-axial joint. Around 50 percent of all movement of the cervical spine occurs at this joint.

From a functional point of view, it's great that we have all of this mobility at the neck. But this can cause problems once we step on the golf course. There, the main thing we really want to do with our head is to keep it still.

The first neck or head issue we usually see involves strength, and it also has its roots in the dysfunctions caused by our 21st-century lifestyle. Standing or sitting upright, your 12-pound head feels pretty weightless because it's balanced comfortably where it's supposed to be. But if we tilt our heads forward a few inches or a few degrees, that all changes. Tilted forward 15 degrees, your head now feels like it weighs around 27 pounds. The farther forward the head gets, the heavier it gets. This would just be mathematical trivia if we walked around all day with good posture and our eyes fixed on the horizon. But we don't. Most of us spend a huge part of our day with our chins intentionally planted in our chests as we glue ourselves to our phones. This

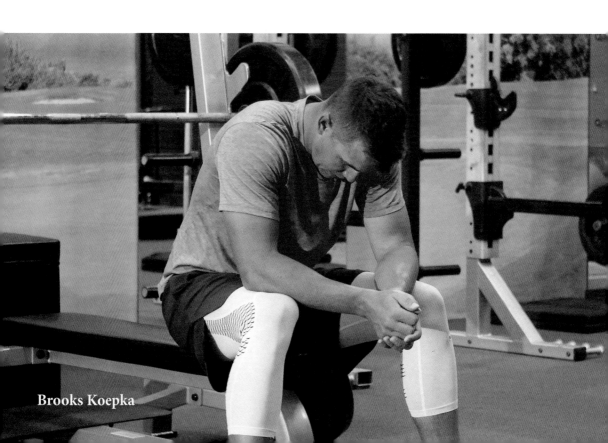

Brooks Koepka

The Anatomy of the Neck & Head

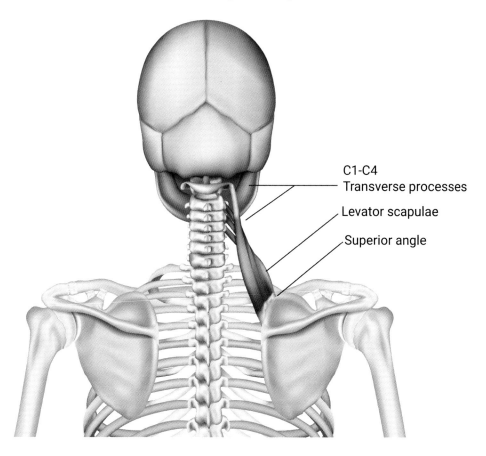

C1-C4
Transverse processes

Levator scapulae

Superior angle

puts an extreme and constant amount of pressure on the muscles that are trying to keep the head upright. And if people's posture was already bad before phones took over our lives, it's only going to get worse.

On the golf course, this postural dysfunction gets multiplied. If there was already a lot of strain on the muscles of the neck and upper back in an upright position, if you have a head-forward posture, things get worse when you try to get into proper golf posture. Now, you've intentionally decided to further tax the already overburdened muscles responsible for keeping your head in the right place.

The Eyes Have It

We've already established the brain and central nervous system's beyond-important role in the golf swing. Based on the sensory feedback it receives, it tells the body exactly what to do in the precise sequence to hit a golf ball. And we've talked about the inner ear's job in helping you stay balanced during your swing. But there's even more inside that 12-pound cranium of yours that's helping you out on the course.

While we're under the impression that we control the movement of our eyes – we look at what we decide to look at, right? – it's a whole lot more complex than that. Think about it. If you're watching a plane fly through the sky, both eyes track the movement of the plane in a similar fashion. Both eyes either track left to right or both eyes track right to left. Similarly, if you're looking out over the green of a par 3 to figure out where you want to land the ball for the safest putt, both eyes scan the green either left to right or right to left.

Now, think about what happens when you're watching someone walk toward you. Both eyes move inward as the person gets closer to you. Now, your right eye is moving to the left and your left eye is moving toward the right in order to track the movement. Similarly, as you line up behind your ball to read a 20-foot putt, your eyes are both focused inward toward the nose as you look at the ball right in front of you, but as your gaze extends forward toward the hole, both eyes track outward – away from the nose – to be able to focus on things farther into the distance.

We've already mentioned the problems that occur in the golf swing if you have a rounded, C-shaped spine. Those same issues with accuracy, consistency, and power will again show up if you have an excessively rounded upper back. In a perfect world, you'd be swinging the club with a relatively straight spine. The more rounded the spine, the less predictable your swing will be. Think about your last home improvement project. It's incredibly easy to screw in a screw that's perfectly straight. Now, imagine how difficult it would be to try to use your screwdriver on a screw with a giant curve in it. You'd end up dealing with a completely unpredictable and chaotic rotation. Think about that the next time you're on the course. Is it more efficient and repeatable to run a straight screw into the wall or a curved one?

If we had to consciously do this every time we tried to look at or focus on anything, we'd be lucky if we could get out of bed in the morning.

The job of performing all of these voluntary and involuntary eye movements falls on six muscles located behind the eyeball. And as you find just about everywhere else in the body, these extraocular muscles come in complementary pairs – one muscle moving the eye in one direction and another muscle moving the eye in the opposing direction.

The lateral rectus and medial rectus are responsible for side-to-side movement of the eyes. The superior rectus and the inferior rectus are responsible for up and down movement. And the superior oblique and inferior oblique muscles aid in diagonal movement of the eyeball.

While the jury is still out as to whether eye exercises can improve declining vision, strengthening the muscles of the eyes – especially if you stare at a lot of screens during the day – can help reduce eye strain and discomfort. (Not unlike how strengthening the muscles of the back and hips can help reduce lower back strain.)

Try alternating your gaze several times between something very close by and something far away. You can also trace a distant skyline with your eyes without moving your head. Alternate between tracing from left to right and tracing from right to left.

Stability issues occur in players who can't control unwanted side-to-side movement of the head during their swing. An optimal golf swing requires perfect rotation around a spine that's fixed in space. We've already talked about the base of the spine when we talked about the hips. Stable hips allow you to lock the base of your spine in place and prevent them from swaying away from – and then toward – your target as you go from address through your backswing through impact and follow-through. That's a good thing, but it's only really half the battle. The head is at the other end of the spine. And your body is going to follow the movement of your head. If your momentum pulls your head away from your target during your backswing, the odds are that you're going to end up in back of your ball at impact.

But having too much movement at the neck and head isn't the only dysfunction that'll negatively affect your game; having too little movement will also add strokes to your score.

We've already talked about the relationship between the lumbar and thoracic spine. And how when each section is allowed to rotate properly, things move very functionally. But when you try to get too much movement where there isn't much movement to be had, there's dysfunction. The key, though, is that these two sections of the spine rotate together in the same direction.

The relationship between the thoracic spine and the cervical spine in the golf swing is even more interesting, because unlike the lower portions of the spine, which needed to work together, the upper portions of the spine have to function independently of each other. Volumes have been written about the importance of the separation between the hips and the shoulders in the golf swing, but just as important is the separation between the head and the shoulders. At the top of your backswing, your shoulders are ideally rotated 90 degrees away from your target, but your head, though, has to stay in a fixed position – facing down with your eyes on the ball.

But what if you don't have the necessary separation between the upper spine and the mid spine? For one thing, your accuracy is going to be very questionable. If you don't have the necessary separation, when you rotate back into your takeaway, not only will that turn rotate your upper body away from the target (which is a good thing), it will also rotate your head and face away from your target (which is a very bad thing). Now, at the top of your backswing, instead of having your eye on the ball, your eyes are now looking at the folks in back of you. As you begin your downswing, you now have to hope that your eyes will be able to find the ball before your club does if you have any chance of hitting things straight.

In slow motion, it might be easy to reestablish eye contact with the ball before your club does, but when you're swinging the club at 100 mph, things are moving pretty fast and you're only going to have a millisecond for your eyes to find your ball. And if you can't lock your eyes onto your ball, you're in trouble. Both accuracy and power will suffer, because the odds of the clubface being where it should be at impact to hit the ball squarely will be awfully low. Another likely scenario is that as you head into your downswing without having eye contact with the ball, you'll start to decelerate to give your eyes more time to find it. Deceleration before impact is a good way to reduce your distance. There needs to be the mobility to create sufficient separation between the head and the shoulders to allow you to get into the top of your backswing without forcing you to take your eyes off the ball.

On the other side of the swing, if you don't have the necessary separation between your upper and mid spine, expect for more dysfunction to occur at impact and into your follow-through. If your head can't maintain its position while the rest of the upper body is rotating, you simply won't be able to keep your eye on your ball at impact. Your head and eyes will essentially be tied to the movement of your chest. Your accuracy will suffer because this is about as close as you can get to swinging with your eyes closed. If, though, you are able to keep your eyes on your ball through impact, it'll mean you're greatly reducing the amount of rotation of your upper body. At this point, you're hitting the ball with a very weak and arms-y swing.

Be aware, not all dysfunctions are symmetrical. You may have adequate separation between the upper and mid spine turning in one direction, but due to any number of reasons, things may feel completely different when you try to turn in the other direction. Movements that improve strength and stability around the neck and head might not be the most impressive exercises you can do at the gym, but they are a surprisingly good way to make solid improvements to your golf game.

Omnidirectional Movement

NECK MOBILITY

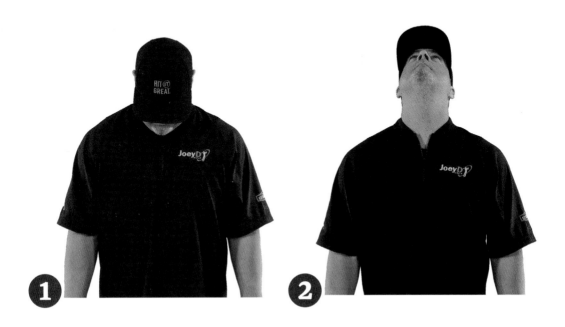

To be able to increase range of motion at the neck – and to check where some asymmetry may exist – try these four simple movements. You may want to perform them in front of a mirror to make it easier to assess any left-side/right-side differences.

1) Stand with feet about shoulder-width apart with strong posture and relaxed shoulders. This is the starting position. Slowly tilt your head as far forward as you can comfortably. Don't force movement if there's discomfort. It should feel like a good stretch in the back of your neck, but there shouldn't be pain. Hold for a three-count.

2) Then, tilt your head as far back as it can go comfortably. You should feel a stretch – but not pain – in the front of your neck across the throat. Hold for a three-count and then return to the starting position. Do five holds in both the forward flexion and backward extension positions.

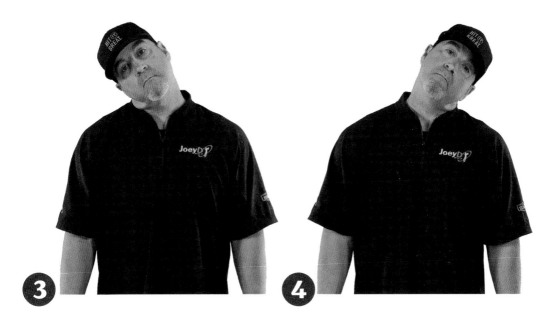

3) From the same starting position, tilt your head to the right side as if you were trying to touch your right ear to your shoulder. Try not to lean or raise your left shoulder. Again, only go as far as you can comfortably. You should feel a stretch on the left side of your neck. Hold for a three-count.

4) Then, tilt your head to the opposite direction, as if you were trying to touch your left ear to your shoulder and hold for a three-count. You should now feel this on the right side of your neck. Do five holds tilting to the right and five holds tilting to the left.

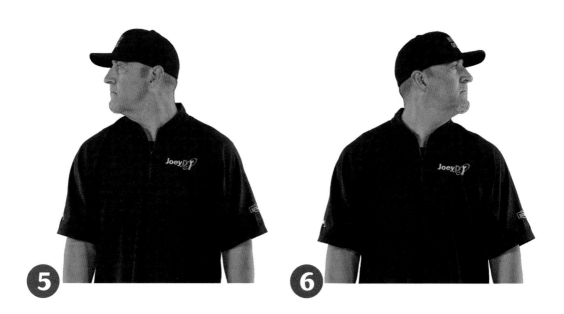

5) Again, from the same starting position and keeping your head perfectly upright, turn your head to the right. Remember to only go as far as feels comfortable. The rest of your body will want to help out on this one, so try to avoid any extra movement at the shoulders and hips. Hold for a three-count.

6) Then, turn your head to the left for a three-count. You may be surprised that you have more freedom of movement in one direction than the other. The ultimate goal is to lessen that difference. Do five holds in each direction.

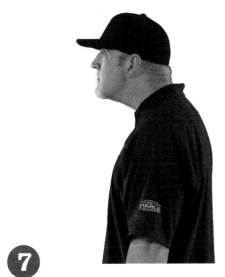

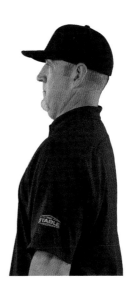

7 **8**

7) Finally, from the same position, jut your head forward keeping your eyes staring straight ahead. If you're using a mirror, keep your eyes on your eyes in your reflection. If you find yourself looking up or down, it means you're tilting your head. Hold this jutted-out position for a three-count and then return to the starting position.

8) Now, pull your head straight back. Imagine you're trying to discreetly distance yourself as much as possible from someone with bad breath. Keep your eyes forward. If you find yourself looking up or down, your head is tilting and you won't be working to increase the targeted range of motion. Hold this for a three-count and return to the starting position. Do five holds in both the jutted-out and the pulled-back position.

Rotation with Eyes on the Ball

NECK STABILITY

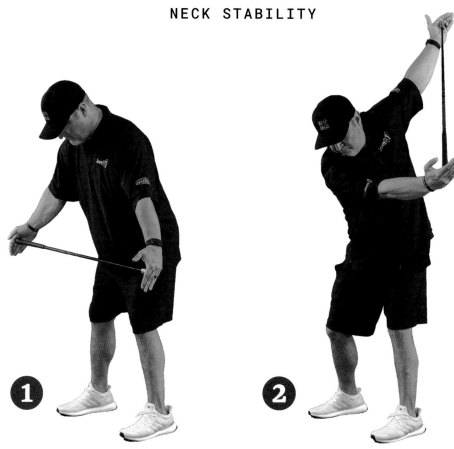

1) Hold a club horizontally in front of you with hands a little bit wider than shoulder-width apart. Assume an address position with good posture and proper spine angle. Fix your eyes on a spot on the floor where your ball would be.

2) From this starting position, rotate to your left into a left-handed player's takeaway position. There'll be a little rotation at the hips, but the majority will be around the spine. The key is to keep your head from turning and keep your eyes fixed on where the ball would be. Hold this position for a beat and then return to your address position.

Now, rotate to your right into a right-handed player's takeaway position. Again, try to keep your head still. Hold for a beat and then return to your address position. Do 10 takeaways in each direction.

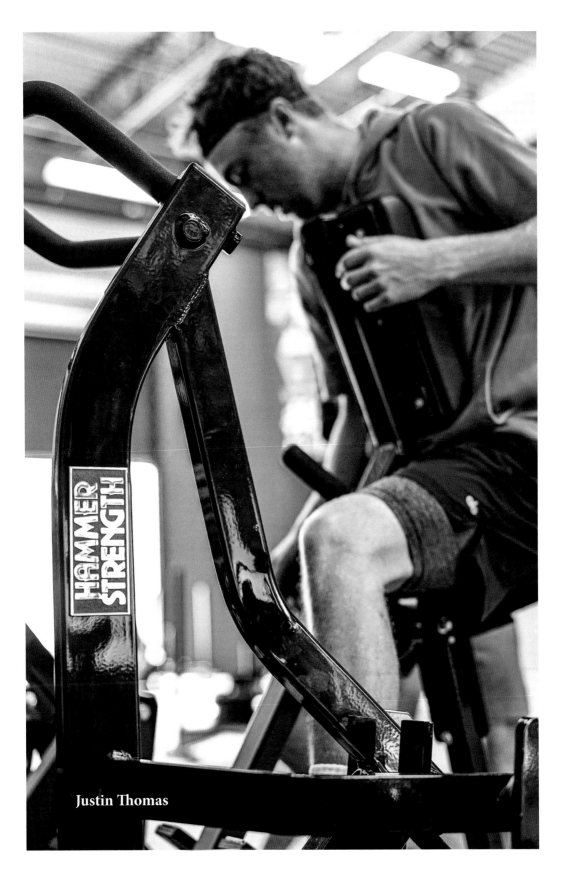

Justin Thomas

Manual Resistance

NECK STRENGTH

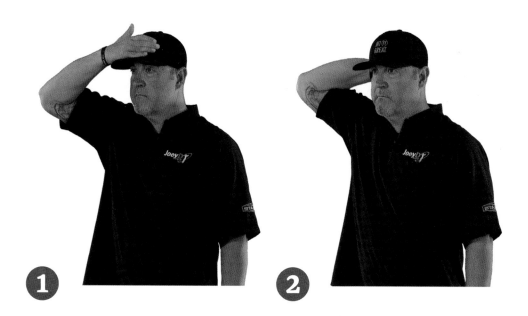

While there's all sorts of equipment and toys available for strengthening the muscles that operate around the neck, two of the safest and most effective ones are your own hands. Stand with feet shoulder-width apart with good posture and relaxed shoulders. You may want to do these movements in front of a mirror to make sure the rest of your body stays quiet.

1) Place the palm of your right hand against your forehead and press gently as if you were trying to tilt your head back. Resist the pressure from your hand and try to keep your head from moving. You may feel this in the muscles in the front of your neck across your throat. This is an example of an isometric contraction. The muscles are engaged, but they're neither shortening (as they usually do when we use them) or lengthening. In an isometric contraction, the muscle maintains its current length. Hold this for a five-count.

2) Now, press gently on the back of your head and use the muscles of the neck to prevent your head from tilting forward. Hold for a five-count.

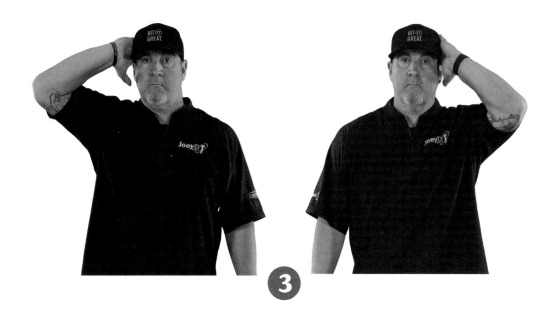

3) Press gently on the right side of your head and resist the pressure to tilt your head to the right. Hold for a five-count and then press on the left side of your head and resist the pressure to tilt your head to the left for a five-count.

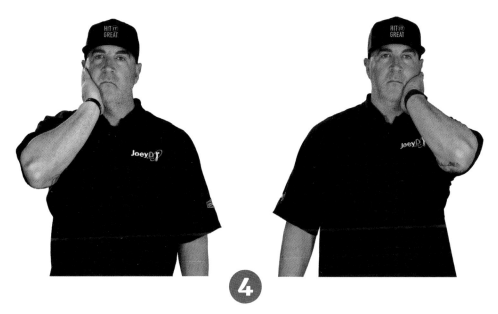

4) Place your palm along your jaw on the right side and press gently. Use the muscles in your neck to prevent your head from turning to the left, and then press gently on the left side of your jaw and resist the pressure to turn your head to the right. Hold both of these for a five-count.

"I'm getting to where my coach wants me to get to in my golf swing, but I think that without the things I'm doing in my workouts, that process would have taken a lot longer."

MARINA ALEX

CHAPTER NINE

The Shoulder

If you've spent any time in the gym, you've probably worked on your shoulders. Strong, powerful, and well-built deltoids – or "delts" – will make you look good. They're the top of the V-shaped back everyone is trying to achieve. The larger your delts are, the more pronounced the taper will be to your waist. Even if you're carrying a little bit of extra weight around your waist, working your delts is a great way to appear slimmer. If the goal of this book was to make you look better in a golf shirt, we'd go on for days about the deltoids, but since you're reading this to help you play better golf, our discussion of the shoulder won't really focus a whole lot on the deltoids.

The shoulders share a lot in common with the hips. The joints are both considered ball-and-socket joints. The hips are where the legs attach to the trunk and the shoulders are where the arms attach to the trunk. Despite the many similarities, there are some significant differences.

The connector between the legs and the spine at the hips is a single bone – the pelvis. The top of the thigh bone fits snugly into a somewhat deep cup in the pelvis, which gives it a lot of stability. At the shoulders, things aren't so simple. Instead of there being one solid bone that things attach to, there are actually three bones. There's the clavicle or collarbone, which you can see and feel running horizontally just above your chest. And there are your shoulder blades, which are made up of your right scapula and left scapula, which you can see and feel in your upper back. This many moving parts allows for an amazing amount of movement, but it also means there's a lot of potential for dysfunction.

For most movements where the arm stays below shoulder height, the top of the upper arm bone – the humerus – sits ball-and-socket-style in a shallow cup in the shoulder blade. The cup is far shallower than the cup in the hip where the leg bone sits. Again, this lets you get away with a lot of movement, but the price you pay is that there's less stability. And that's only half the problem. When the arm is raised above shoulder height, the outer tip of the collarbone is required to help hold the top of the humerus in place. Now, things are even less stable than when the arm was lower than shoulder height – and that wasn't all that stable to begin with!

While big muscles like the deltoids, the pectorals (the large muscles of the chest), and the latissimus dorsi (the large muscle of the back) help stabilize a lot that goes on around the shoulder, the main stabilizers of the shoulder are the four muscles that make up the rotator cuff – the supraspinatus, infraspinatus, teres minor, and subscapularis.

Thanks for putting up with about 500 words of physiology and anatomy, but it's these four rotator cuff muscles that we're most concerned with.

You don't need massive delts, pecs, and lats to play golf. In fact, we've already talked about how overly tight lats or pecs may negatively affect your ability to create proper spine angle and maintain a strong golf posture. The muscles of the rotator cuff are another story. Properly functioning rotators are vital to the golf swing. And when it comes to the muscles of the rotator cuff, you need both strength and sufficient range of motion.

But what exactly is shoulder rotation?

Raise your arm out to the side or in front of you and then turn your palm up. Now turn your palm down. You've just created rotation at the shoulder.

With your arm by your side, flex your elbow to 90 degrees so that your forearm is parallel to the floor and your fingers are pointing forward. Now, while keeping your upper arm tight against your body, turn your forearm so that it's flat against the front of your body. You've just created internal rotation at the shoulder.

Raise your arm out to the side so that it's parallel to the floor. Bend your elbow

The Anatomy of the Shoulder

A DETAIL OF THE SHOULDER AREA

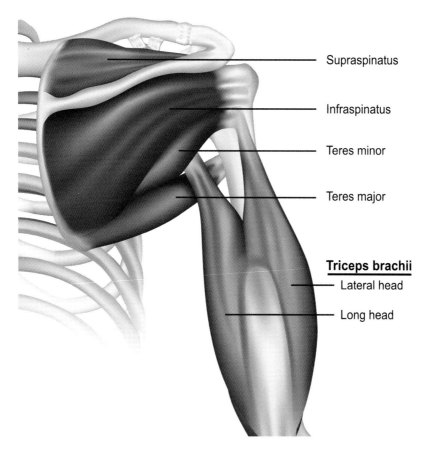

Supraspinatus

Infraspinatus

Teres minor

Teres major

Triceps brachii
Lateral head

Long head

90 degrees keeping the forearm parallel to the floor. Now, without moving your upper arm, raise your forearm until it's vertical and perpendicular to the floor – as if you were testifying in court. You've just created external rotation at the shoulder.

When we talked about the role of the hips and spine in the golf swing, we mentioned the high possibility of injury due to either weakness, tightness, or improper technique. The good news about the shoulders is that it's rare that someone develops a shoulder injury from playing golf. The bad news is that if you've had a previous shoulder injury that never quite healed properly, it may have a negative impact on your game.

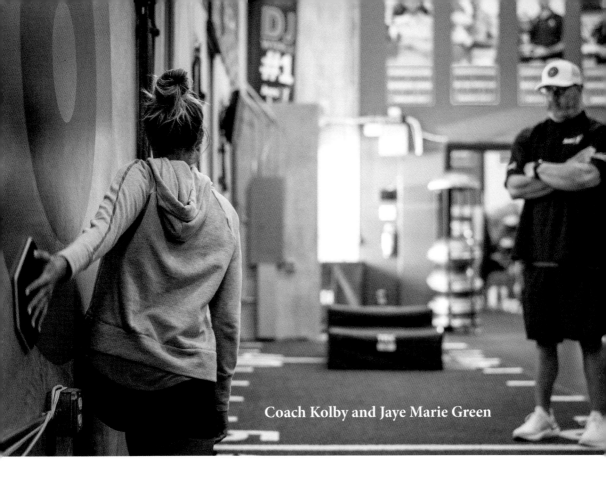

Coach Kolby and Jaye Marie Green

A lot of the postural issues that we've already discussed can be attributed to our current, more sedentary lifestyles. They're injuries that owe more to inactivity than activity. Shoulder issues generally are due to overactivity. Shoulder injuries to athletes usually come from overuse – throwing a baseball, serving a tennis ball, swimming. Similarly, non-sports shoulder injuries also can come from overuse or chronic misuse – spending eight hours a day cutting hair, doing overhead construction work, etc.

Because of this, we see a lot of shoulder issues. Many golfers didn't start playing the game until they were no longer able to play another sport due to an injury. And a lot of the time, the injury they suffered was a shoulder injury.

If there's limited range of rotational motion at the shoulder, it will affect your golf swing. Just as with the hips, there needs to be sufficient amounts of internal and external rotation at the shoulders to properly move the club. If you're a right-handed player, you need to be able to keep the upper part of your right arm against your body and externally rotate the forearm as you begin your takeaway. If your body won't allow you to externally rotate properly, you'll generally end up compensating by lifting your entire arm away from your body. Once you've gone into this chicken wing position – and look like a baseball player holding a golf club – your chances of maintaining a proper swing plane are pretty slim.

Even if you have the discipline to keep your right arm tight by your side during your takeaway, if there's limited external rotation in your right shoulder, there are still a couple of things that you need to be aware of. First off, you're just not going to get as full of a backswing as you'd want. It's great that you have the body control not to let your arm chicken wing out, but if you can't get sufficient external rotation, your backswing is going to be very limited. Power comes from maximizing clubhead speed at impact. If your downswing is shortened due to a limited backswing, your power – and your distance – will suffer.

And if you're able to keep your right arm tight by your side, but are appalled at your measly takeaway and feel the need to look exactly like the guys on TV and in the magazines, you're going to go into an excessive lean to get the club to where you think it needs to be. Now, you're starting your downswing from an off-balanced, front-leaning position. Being off-balance is an interesting human condition. When you're off-balance, subconsciously all you really want to do is regain your equilibrium. All that careful planning and mathematical calculations based on the distance to your target, the width of the fairway, and the wind speed and direction go right out the window. Hitting the ball properly is no longer your body's prime concern. All your body wants to do is keep itself from falling over. So, what happens? You start to decelerate far too early. You may end up hitting the ball, but because of your shaky balance and slower clubhead speed, both your power and accuracy will be sacrificed.

On the other side of your swing, if you don't have the ability to externally rotate your left arm after impact and into your follow-through, you're looking at more issues. Because you don't have the range of motion to comfortably finish with a deep follow-through, subconsciously, you'll start to decelerate your swing prematurely in order to stay in balance. As we just mentioned – and as we've mentioned plenty of other times, as well – decelerating your swing early will result in a loss of power at impact.

How do you know if you have sufficient external rotation? Here's a simple assessment that you can do based on a movement we just described.

Stand with your back against a wall with your arms out to the side at shoulder height. Bend your elbows 90 degrees so that your forearms are still at shoulder height and parallel to the floor, but now your fingers are pointing forward. Your upper arm should still be fully connected to the wall. Keeping your upper arm against the wall, slowly rotate your right forearm upward so that it's perpendicular to the floor and your fingers are pointing to the ceiling. The goal is to get your forearm to fully connect with the wall. (Be aware that your lower back may want to move away from the wall to allow the forearm to move more. Don't let that happen!) Return the right forearm to the starting position and try the same movement with your left forearm.

If you were able to make full contact with the wall with your forearm, you have a good amount of external rotation. If not, don't fret. Most people – even those that go to the gym regularly – don't do things to strengthen and increase rotational range of motion around the shoulders. But by focusing on stretching and strengthening these smaller muscles in the shoulder, you'll be amazed not only at how much you'll improve your ability to externally rotate the shoulder, but also how much easier, effortless, and powerful your golf swing will become.

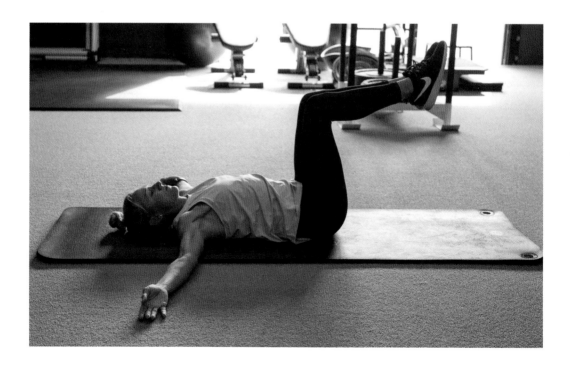

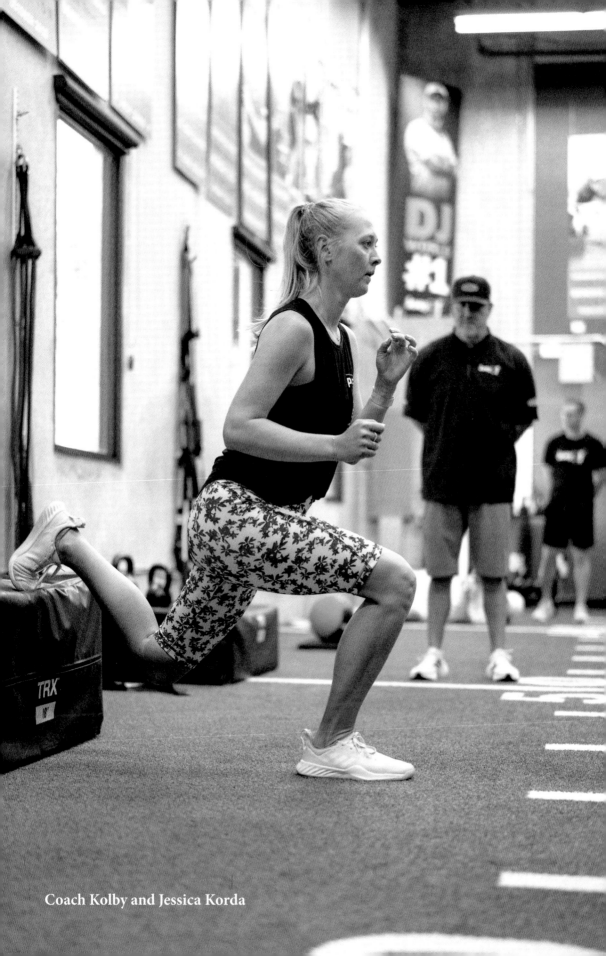

Coach Kolby and Jessica Korda

Forearm Slides

SHOULDER STABILITY

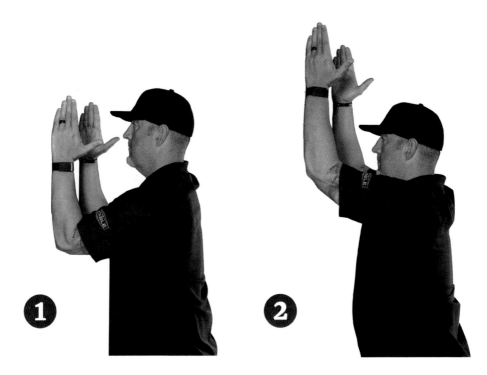

1) To create stability at the shoulder, stand facing a wall. Your feet should be about a foot from the base of the wall. Place your forearms vertically against the wall with your palms facing in toward each other. In this position, just your pinkie fingers should be in contact with the wall with your thumbs pointing toward your ears. Your elbows should be just below chest level and your hands should be about at the same height as your face. This is the starting position.

2) Slowly, keeping your forearms vertical and in contact with the wall, slide them upward. Keep sliding until your arms are straight. Hold this for a moment and then, keeping your forearms vertical and in contact with the wall, reverse the movement until you're back to the starting position.

If one or both shoulders don't have adequate stability, you might find it difficult to maintain constant contact with the wall or to keep your forearms vertical. You might also find that your shoulders move way up toward your ears. If any of these compensations were an issue, reduce the range of motion of the movement until you can do a limited version of this movement without any compensations. Over time, you'll be able to create greater range of motion and you'll find that you're doing the movement with far less stress in the shoulders. Try for 10 slides without any compensations to complete the set.

Progression: Perform the previous movement with a light-resistance looped band around your forearms right above the elbow. There should be light tension in the band at the starting position of the move. If there's any instability, it will become obvious immediately, as your forearms will either angle in toward each other or they'll come away from the wall. Again, as previously mentioned, if you're able to do a limited range version of this without any compensations, perform the limited range version until the stabilizers in the shoulders become strong enough to complete the full range version. Whether there were any compensations or not, you may be feeling this exercise in places that you've never felt anything before. Congrats! You've discovered some new body parts!

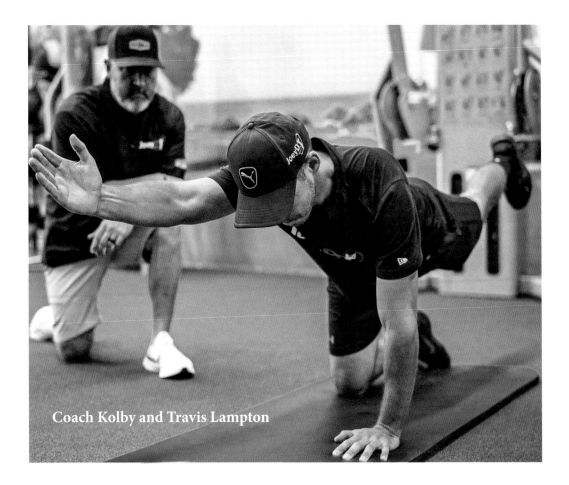

Coach Kolby and Travis Lampton

Internal Rotation
with Band

SHOULDER MOBILITY

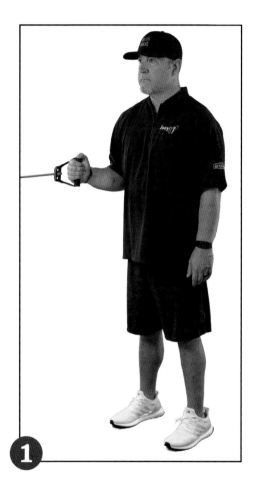
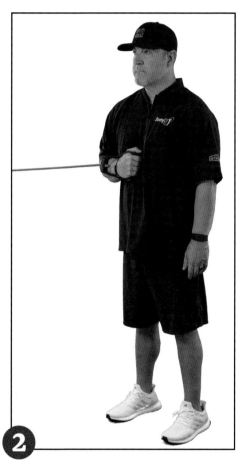

1) As we've discussed, limited ability to rotate the shoulder will negatively affect your game in a major way. To strengthen the muscles that rotate the shoulders internally, stand sideways to the anchor point of a light resistance band set between waist and chest height. The right side of your body should be facing the anchor point, and you should have the band handle in your right hand. Press your upper arm tight against your body and flex your elbow 90 degrees. With the band handle in your hand, the back of your hand should be facing the anchor point. This is the starting position.

2) Keeping your hips, chest, and shoulders squared forward and your upper arm against your body, rotate your forearm away from the anchor point and across your body. There are many keys to doing this one correctly, but the main one is to make sure the rotation happens in a true horizontal plane and that your forearm stays parallel to the floor the entire time. If it's not moving in a parallel plane, you're not targeting the rotators. (For example, if you're moving at a slightly upward angle, you're actually doing a strange version of a biceps curl, and if you're moving at a slightly downward angle, you're allowing your triceps to get involved.) You also want to prevent your arm from coming away from your body. A good way to prevent this is to place a folded towel under your arm between your upper arm and your body. If the towel falls to the floor, you'll know that you've lost contact.

Hold this forearm-across-your-body position for a three-count and then return to the starting position in a controlled manner to complete the rep. You may find that it's incredibly easy to do the move with one arm, but that it's far more difficult with the other. The goal, as it is with everything we're doing, is to reduce whatever asymmetry exists. Shoot for 10 reps with each arm.

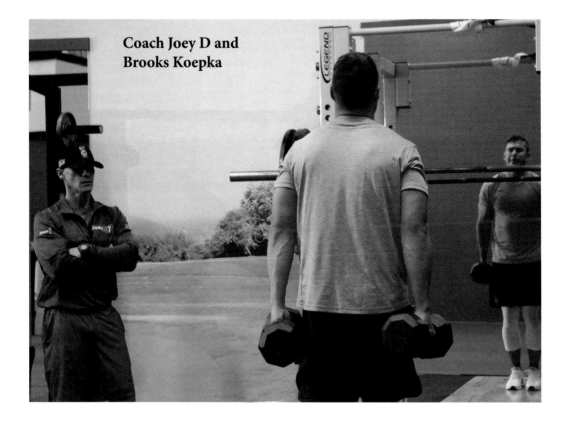

Coach Joey D and
Brooks Koepka

External Rotation with Band

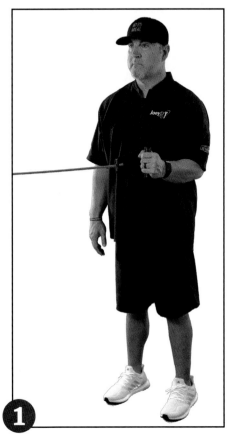 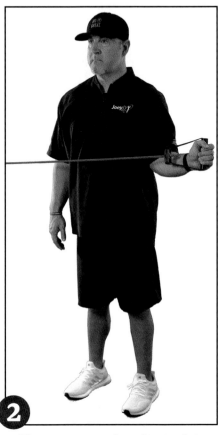

Limited external rotation will affect your golf even more than limited internal rotation, so it's vital to target your external rotators. The external rotators don't generate as much force as the internal rotators, so you want to go with a lighter resistance band for this one or stand a little bit closer to the anchor point.

1) Position yourself as you did in the previous exercise with a band handle in your left hand, your upper arm pressed tight against your body, and your elbow flexed at 90 degrees with your forearm parallel to the floor. The right side of your body and the palm of your left hand should both be facing the anchor point. Let the tension of the band pull your forearm toward the anchor point without letting it pull your upper arm away from your body. This is the starting point.

2) Keeping your hips, chest, and shoulders squared forward and your upper arm against your body, rotate your forearm away from the anchor point as if your forearm was a door opening. Hold this position for a three-count and then slowly reverse the move and return to the starting position in a controlled manner with your forearm staying parallel to the floor to complete the rep.

Because the external rotators aren't as strong as the internal rotators, there are going to be a whole lot of potential compensations to be aware of. As in the previous move, make sure that you move the forearm in a perfectly horizontal plane to avoid recruiting the biceps and triceps. More importantly, though, be aware that your entire body is going to want to help your left hand get that band handle from point A to point B. Be very aware not to let your hips, chest, or shoulders rotate to the left and away from the anchor point. This is a very big red flag that indicates lack of strength in the external rotators. What's nice about using bands for this exercise is that it's very easy to reduce the resistance in the band just by moving a few inches closer to the anchor point, so you may end up doing this movement with less tension in the band for one arm than for the other. Over time, these right-side/left-side imbalances will become reduced or disappear entirely. Again, do 10 reps with each arm.

Single-Arm Flies
with Band

CHEST STRENGTH AT THE SHOULDER

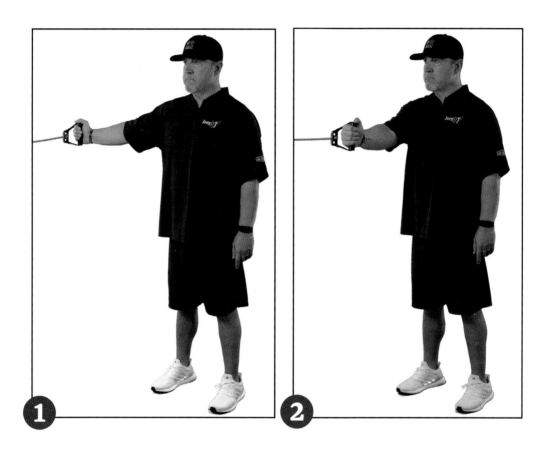

A great chest exercise that will not only strengthen and stretch your pecs in a golf-specific way, but will also help shore up the infrastructure of the shoulder.

1) With a band handle in your right hand, stand with feet shoulder-width apart with the band anchor point in back of and to the right of you. Extend your right arm directly out to the side with a slight bend at your elbow. Your right hand should now be directly in front of the anchor point with your palm facing forward and there should be tension in the band. Your hips, chest, and shoulders should be squared forward, and your upper body should be upright with good posture. This is the starting point.

2) Keeping the rest of your body still and quiet and maintaining a slight bend at the elbow, draw your arm forward until it's extended directly in front of you. The movement should happen in a horizontal plane parallel to the floor and it should involve movement only at the shoulder. You should not only feel this in your chest and shoulder, but because of the imbalances that are being created by the one-sidedness of the movement, you should also feel it in the core, hips, and legs. Hold this position for a second and then slowly reverse the move to return to the starting position. To get the most out of this exercise, don't simply let the tension of the band pull you back to the starting position. Resist the tension and return to the starting position in a controlled fashion. Do 10 flies with each arm to complete the set.

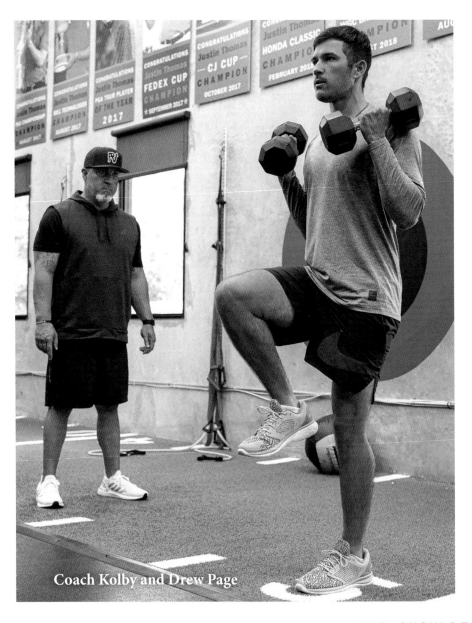

Coach Kolby and Drew Page

Shoulder Blade Retraction with Bands

RHOMBOID STRENGTH AT THE SHOULDER

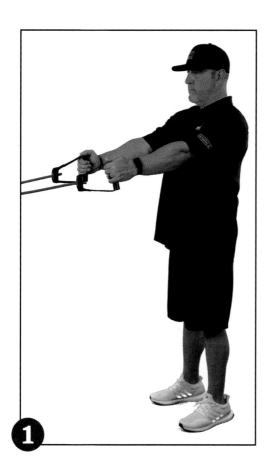

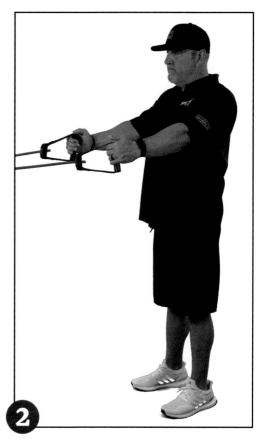

Strengthening deep postural muscles like the rhomboids aren't what most people think of when it comes to a shoulder workout, but you're working to optimize your body for golf, not a mixed martial arts fight in the Octagon. This is a great one for improving your ability to maintain good golf posture and spine angle. It's also a move that most people have never done in isolation, so it may take a while to get used to. Once you do get a feel for the movement, though, you'll feel taller every time you do it!

1) Stand facing a band anchor point set at shoulder height with a band handle in each hand. Straighten your arms toward the anchor point. There should be slight tension in the bands. This is the starting point.

2) Moving just your arms, pull back your shoulders by squeezing your shoulder blades together. This isn't a big movement. Your arms will retract a total of six to eight inches. But, again, this one might be tough at first. If you find your elbows bending, it's because your body is going to want to use the big muscles in the back and turn this into a pulling motion. You also may find yourself leaning backward to move your shoulders back. Avoid either of these compensations. When you've drawn the band back as far as you can comfortably go, hold the position for a three-count before letting the arms return back toward the anchor point to complete the rep.

If the move seems too foreign and difficult using the bands, try it without the bands and just try to isolate the drawing back and squeezing of your shoulder blades while keeping your arms straight. Once you're able to do this comfortably and with good control, try it again with the bands. Do 10 repetitions with proper form.

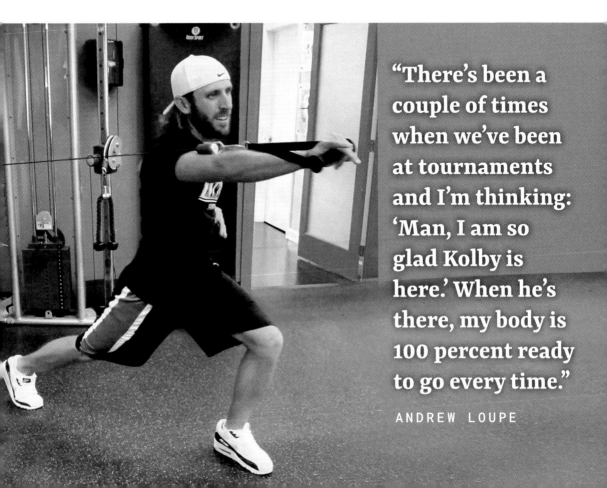

"There's been a couple of times when we've been at tournaments and I'm thinking: 'Man, I am so glad Kolby is here.' When he's there, my body is 100 percent ready to go every time."

ANDREW LOUPE

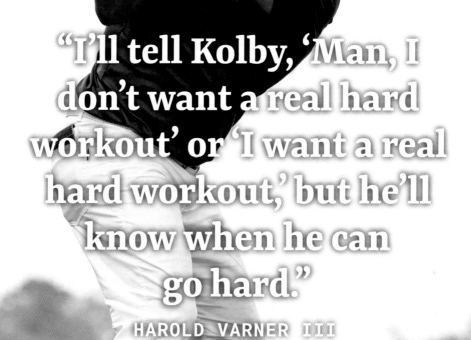

"I'll tell Kolby, 'Man, I don't want a real hard workout' or 'I want a real hard workout,' but he'll know when he can go hard."

HAROLD VARNER III

CHAPTER TEN

The Elbow

When it comes to the elbow's role in the golf swing, most folks think they can sum it up in three words: keep it tucked. And while it's true that if you're a right-handed golfer, keeping your right elbow tucked as you initiate your takeaway is a big key to a successful swing, the elbow's role in the golf swing is far bigger. And dysfunction at the elbow could be costing you strokes and causing you pain.

Structurally, the elbow shares a lot in common with the knee. They're both hinge-style joints. But while movement at the knee is essentially limited to flexion and extension – you can bend your leg and you can straighten your leg – the design of the elbow allows for a little more movement.

With your arms by your side, flex your elbow 90 degrees so that your forearms are parallel to the floor and your palms are facing up. Keeping your arms tight against your sides, turn your hands so that your palms are now facing down. Now turn them so that your palms are facing up again. You've just created rotational movement at the elbow. Pronation is when you turn your palms toward the floor and supination is when you turn your palms toward the ceiling. If you had done that same movement with your arms fully outstretched in front of you – without the bend in the elbow – the rotation would have originated at the shoulder, as we detailed in the previous chapter.

The muscle groups responsible for flexion and extension – or bending and straightening the arm – are familiar to most people. Your biceps on the front of your upper arm create flexion and your triceps on the back of your upper arm create extension and are responsible for straightening the arm. And it's our obsession with these muscles – especially the biceps – that leads to a common dysfunction that we see.

Back when we were first introducing the concept of species-specific training and examining how pairs of muscles work as partners, we gave the example of someone who primarily focused on their biceps in their workouts and didn't spend equal time on their triceps. The result was that the biceps were chronically shortened and that the triceps were chronically lengthened. In simpler terms, the result of this unbalanced workout left the person unable to completely straighten their arms.

So, what happens out on the course if you can't straighten your arms? For one thing, there's going to be the tendency to chicken wing the elbow in both your takeaway and follow-through, which will affect both ends of your swing. Second, shortening the combined length of your arm and club by not being able to fully extend the arms will steal clubhead speed, power, and distance from your swing.

Earlier, we mentioned the importance of keeping the combined length of your arm and club as long as possible – or why for maximum clubhead speed, power, and distance, you want to make contact with the arms fully extended. To help explain some of the physics behind this, think back to when you were a kid putting those green army men on an LP record while it was playing. Sure, it wasn't the most audiophile thing you could have done, but it did teach you something about centrifugal force – even if you didn't know it at the time. The guys you put near the inner part of the record were able to stand up proudly while the guys you put near the edge of the record generally ended up flying off the album and would have been considered collateral damage. The farther something is from the point of rotation, be it the spindle in the center of your turntable or your spine in the golf swing, the faster it moves. The farther away your clubhead is during your swing, the faster it will move. And more clubhead speed at impact means more power and distance.

All things being equal, an ideal swing with full arm extension will have more clubhead speed at impact then the same swing with less than full extension. It's also a main reason why golf favors taller players – especially if those guys have long arms. A Dustin Johnson at 6'3" is just structurally better suited to hitting a ball long than, say, Brian Harman is at 5'7". Harman can do other things to lengthen his game and DJ might be doing things inadvertently to shorten his game, but – from a purely biomechanical point of view – longer arms will hit the ball farther. So, if you're a shorter player, in addition to making sure that you're generating as much power as possible through the legs and hips, a big key to hitting it long is being able to get full arm extension at impact.

The Anatomy of the Elbow

A DETAIL OF THE JOINT, TENDONS, AND MUSCLES

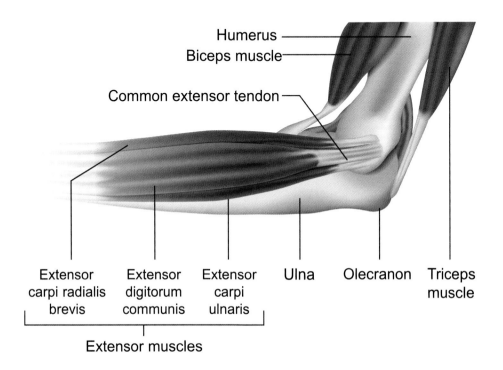

Humerus
Biceps muscle
Common extensor tendon
Extensor carpi radialis brevis
Extensor digitorum communis
Extensor carpi ulnaris
Ulna
Olecranon
Triceps muscle
Extensor muscles

"I'm not a very big person – I'm like 5'3" or 5'4" – so for me getting speed and power has always been a little bit of a struggle. I just don't have that natural strength or height. So, these are the things we work on in the gym." – Marina Alex

Need more convincing to be less biceps-obsessed in the gym?

For one thing, the triceps make up about two-thirds of the size of your upper arm, so if you're just shooting to look good in short sleeves, you definitely don't want to be ignoring your triceps. And second, on the golf course, the triceps are far more important to the swing than the biceps. It's the triceps' job to straighten the arm and to keep it straight against resistance. If your clubhead is traveling at 100-plus mph during your downswing, you need strong triceps to keep your arms straight and fully extended at impact.

Tight biceps and lack of flexion at the elbow aren't the only conditions that can affect your swing. Hypermobility can also be a problem. A lot of people can not only fully straighten their arms, but they can also extend them beyond what would be considered a normal range of motion. Put simply, people with hypermobility at the elbow have the ability to bend their arms in what most people would consider "the wrong direction." This can lead to instability issues at the elbow that can result in power and accuracy issues on the course. To minimize the impact of hypermobility – and to prevent potential injury – there needs to be added focus on the balance between biceps strength and triceps strength. Again, the goal is full extension of the arms at impact.

The elbow isn't just about flexion and extension. The ability to create rotation is the primary feature of the elbow joint that's missing from the knee joint. You simply can't rotate your lower leg until the bottom of your foot is facing up. (Go ahead. Give it a try!) Remember, though, regardless of what joint we're talking about, increased mobility comes at the cost of decreased stability. So, while the ability to rotate the forearm lets you do everything from turning a doorknob and using a screwdriver to pouring coffee and drinking from a glass, it does open you up for creating dysfunction.

Golfer's elbow is a painful condition caused by the repetitive motion of the golf swing coupled with less-than-optimal form and weakness in the muscles of the forearm – including one of the primary rotators of the wrist. It's generally felt on or around the bony nub on the inner side of the elbow. The rotator muscle that attaches there is responsible for turning the palm downward. On the golf course, this turning-the-palm-down happens every time you turn your wrists through impact. If the muscles responsible for this very repetitive movement aren't strong enough to deal with the amount of work they need to do, they will complain. And if you're someone who chunks the ball every once in a while, this puts an amazing amount of strain on the forearm that you'll feel in the elbow.

In extreme cases of injury or dysfunction, the ligament on the inner part of the elbow may actually get damaged. In this case, surgery is needed. Ulnar collateral ligament reconstruction is better known as Tommy John surgery – named after the baseball pitcher whose career was revived after undergoing the procedure. The surgery is far more common among baseball pitchers than golfers. (And the jury is still out as to whether or not it's cool to have a medical procedure named after you.)

Golfer's elbow is similar to – but in some ways the opposite of – tennis elbow. Tennis elbow is a painful condition that affects the outer part of the elbow and involves the muscles on the back of the forearm – including the muscles responsible for turning the palm up. Very few people head to the gym planning to work on the muscles that flip the palm over and back, but if you're a golfer, a tennis player, or both, you need to be working on these functionally important rotator muscles.

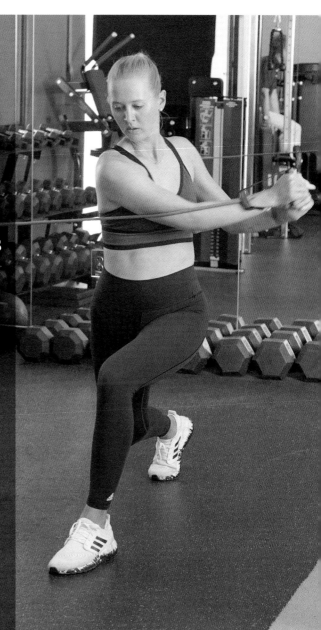

"I'm double-jointed and hypermobile, so we have to get a little more creative with what we do. I have 25 degrees of hyperextension in my left elbow and 15 degrees in my right elbow. For every exercise, we have to pay attention to what my 'normal' is. It's not just about building muscle. A lot of it is injury prevention. And if something is hurting, we're able to fix it."

JESSICA KORDA

Biceps Stretch

ELBOW MOBILITY

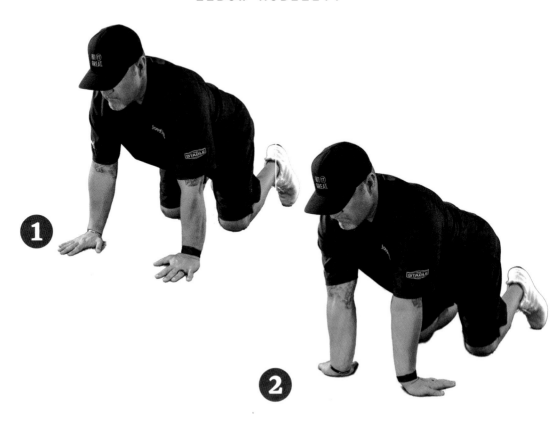

This is a great move for stretching into the biceps and creating more range of motion at the elbow. If you've never stretched your biceps before, this one will feel pretty interesting.

1) Get onto all fours on the ground with your wrists aligned directly under your shoulders and your knees directly aligned under your hips. If you did this the way 99 percent of the population would, your fingers of both hands are pointing forward with your palms on the ground.

2) Carefully rotate your arms to try to get your fingers facing out to the sides with your palms on the floor. Now gently press your elbows inward and toward each other as you straighten your arms as much as possible. You should feel a deep stretch into both your biceps and the front of your forearms. Hold the stretch for 20 seconds. Do three 20-second holds with a 20-second break in between each to complete the set.

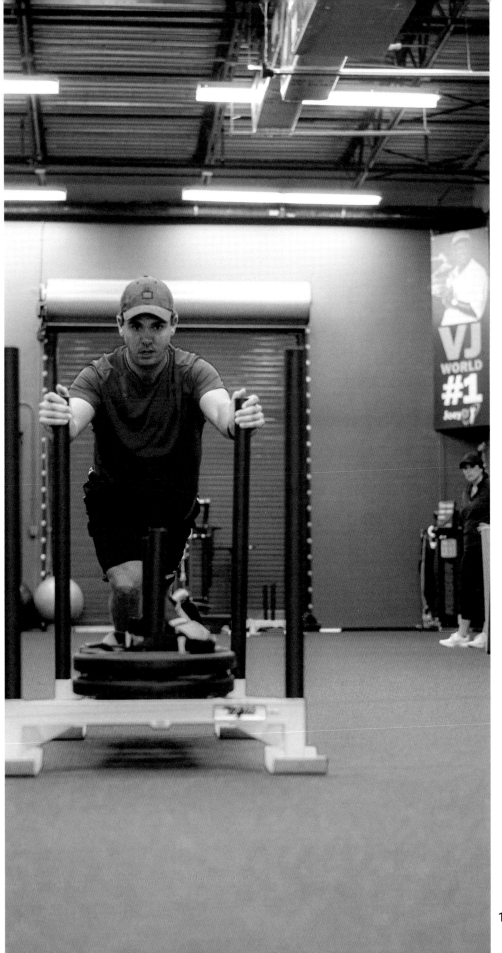

Straight Arm Planks

ELBOW STABILITY

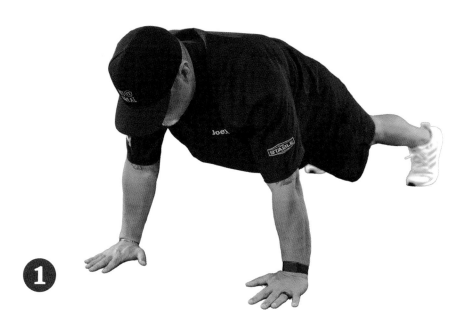

A great way to increase stability at the elbow and shoulders while also challenging your entire core.

1) Assume an "up" push-up position with your hands aligned directly under your shoulders. Your body should be in a straight line from the top of your head to your heels. This is the position you're shooting for. You may want to do this using a mirror so that you can see a sideways view of your body.

Hold the plank position only so long as you can without either of the above compensations becoming too powerful to correct. Shoot initially for three 10-second holds for each set and work your way up to three 20-second holds per set.

A bunch of things are going to want to happen. Your hips are going to want to drop and your lower back is going to want to arch. This is a sign of weak glutes. Curl your hips under to prevent this from happening. When you do, you should feel your glutes engaging and your body straightening. This corrective move is essentially the same hip movement that you did in the Cat/Cow mobility exercise from the Spine chapter.

The other thing to look for and to try to avoid is having your body pike and your butt raise up in the air. This is the sign of a weak core. Drop your hips and engage your abdominal muscles to realign your body into a straight line.

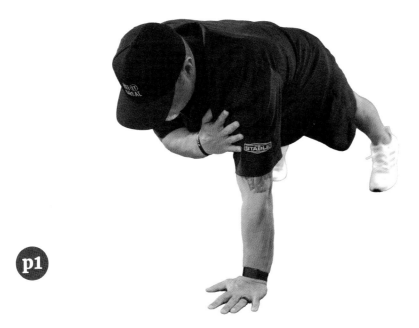

Progression One: From the same starting plank position, challenge the stability at the elbow and shoulder even more by taking your right hand off the floor and bringing it to your left shoulder. Hold for a five-count and then return it to the floor. Now bring your left hand to your right shoulder for a five-count. The unsupported shoulder is going to want to drop. Try not to let this happen. Also, try not to let the other two compensations discussed above happen.

Initially, for each set, shoot for three planks with two alternating holds on each side and eventually work your way up three planks where you're able to do five alternating holds on each side.

Triceps Extensions

TRICEPS STRENGTH AT THE ELBOW

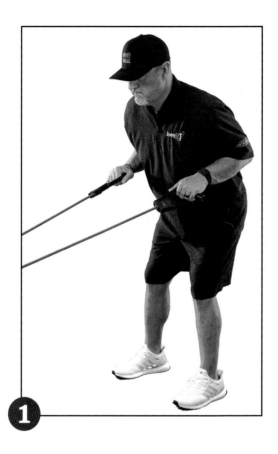

1) This is a great move for strengthening the back of the upper arm and lessening any biceps/triceps muscular imbalances that may exist. Stand facing a band anchor point set at chest height with a band handle in each hand. Assume a comfortable address position with knees bent, shoulders relaxed, and with good posture and spine angle. Bring your upper arms tight against your sides and flex your elbows so that the bands and your forearms are in a perfectly straight line from the anchor point to your elbows. Turn your palms down, so that they're facing the floor. This is the starting position.

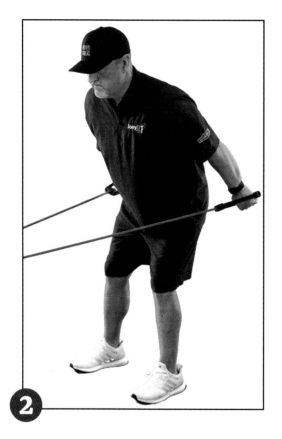

2) Keeping your upper arms tight against your sides and your palms facing down, straighten your arms by moving only at the elbow. At the end of the movement, your arms should be as straight as you can get them with your hands now in back of you with your palms facing up. You should feel this in the back of your upper arms, but because of the added stability requirements of being in golf posture, you may feel this in the lower back, hips, and legs. If you're unable to do the move without your upper arm moving, move a few inches closer to the anchor point. Hold this position for a second and then reverse the movement to return to the starting position to complete the rep. And to get the most out of this move, it's just as important that the upper arm remains glued to your side during the return phase of the exercise as it is during the initial phase. Shoot for 10 reps with good form.

Progression One: From the same starting position, perform the same move as on the previous page, but now alternate the movements so that as one arm is straightening away from the anchor point, the other arm is flexing back toward the anchor point. This will add a few interesting, challenging, and beneficial wrinkles to the exercise. In the original move, there was exertion, a static hold, a slow return, and then a rest period. Here, there's constant motion. There's also a slight increase in the full-body stability needed to maintain proper golf posture as both arms are constantly moving in opposite directions. As a result, this one may get your heart rate up a little faster and you may feel more of a burn in your triceps. Do 10 alternating reps with each arm to complete the set.

Progression Two: As long as we're throwing some chaos at you, let's turn the knob even more. This time perform the progression above, but while standing on two balance pads. Now, we've opened up the gates for a lot to go wrong. The added full-body stability required to deal with the alternating arm movements gets increased further by your need to maintain proper posture and spine angle while balancing on unstable surfaces. And don't let the added balance challenge distract you from the primary focus of the move. Make sure to keep your upper arms by your side throughout the entire move to force your triceps to do as much work as possible. As with the above progression, shoot for 10 reps with each arm.

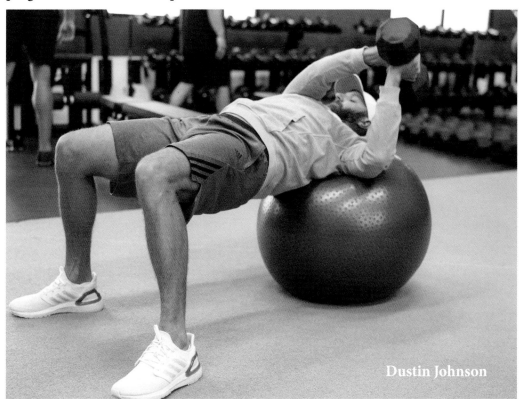

Dustin Johnson

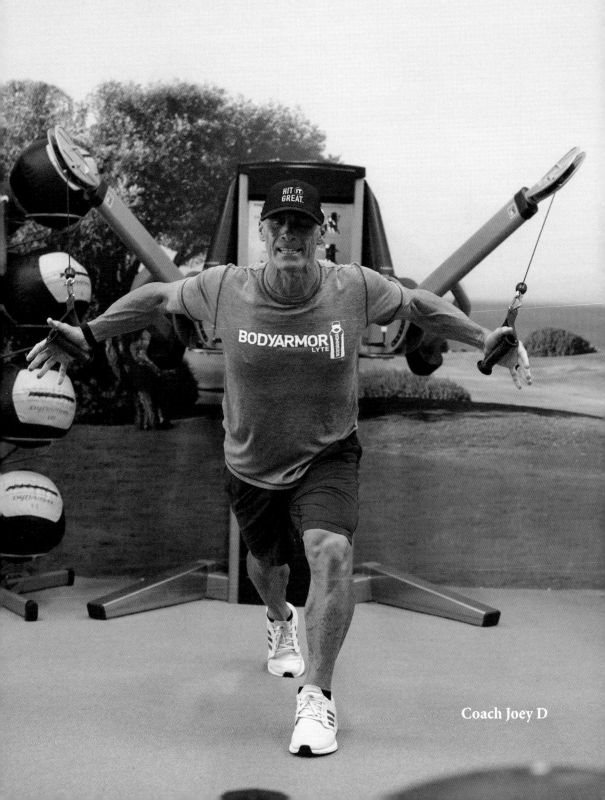

Coach Joey D

Wrist Pronation
with Band

FOREARM STRENGTH AT THE ELBOW

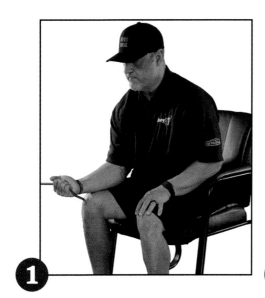

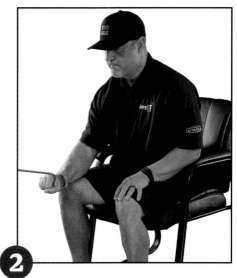

1) To strengthen the muscles that help you turn your wrists over and to help prevent golfer's elbow, sit comfortably on a bench or a chair with a band anchor point directly to your right set at slightly higher than knee height. Your feet should be slightly wider than hip-width apart with your feet flat on the ground. Grab the band – not the handle – with your right hand and place your right forearm on your right thigh. Your fist should be extended slightly past your knee with your palm facing the ceiling. In this position, the anchor point should be on the same side as your thumb. Hold your right forearm in place with your left hand to prevent any unnecessary movement. This is the starting position.

2) Holding the band tightly and without letting your forearm move, turn your fist so that your palm is now facing the floor. Hold for a three-count and then slowly reverse the move to return to the starting position to complete the repetition. Make sure to keep your forearm quiet and stable as you return to the starting position. Go with a relatively light resistance band for this one to make sure that you're able to perform the move without any compensations. For each set, do 10 reps with each arm.

Wrist Supination with Band

FOREARM STRENGTH AT THE ELBOW

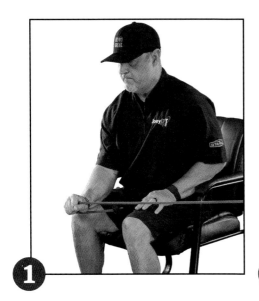 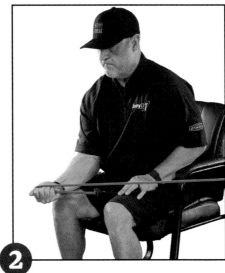

1) To work the forearm muscles responsible for turning the wrist and hand in the opposite and upward facing direction, assume the same starting position, but this time have the anchor point set up on your left side at slightly higher than knee height. With the band in your right hand – again, the band, not the handle – place your forearm against your thigh with your palm facing the floor. In this position, the anchor point should again be on the same side as your thumb. Use your left hand to brace and stabilize your right forearm. This is the starting position.

2) Without moving your forearm, turn your fist over until your palm is now facing the ceiling. Hold this position for a three-count and then reverse the movement while keeping the forearm from moving to complete the rep. Don't let the tension in the band pull you back to the starting position. Slowly return to the starting position to get the most out of the movement. Again, you're going to want to go with a lighter resistance band to make sure that you can do the exercise without any compensations or extra movement. As with the previous exercise, do 10 reps with each arm to complete the set.

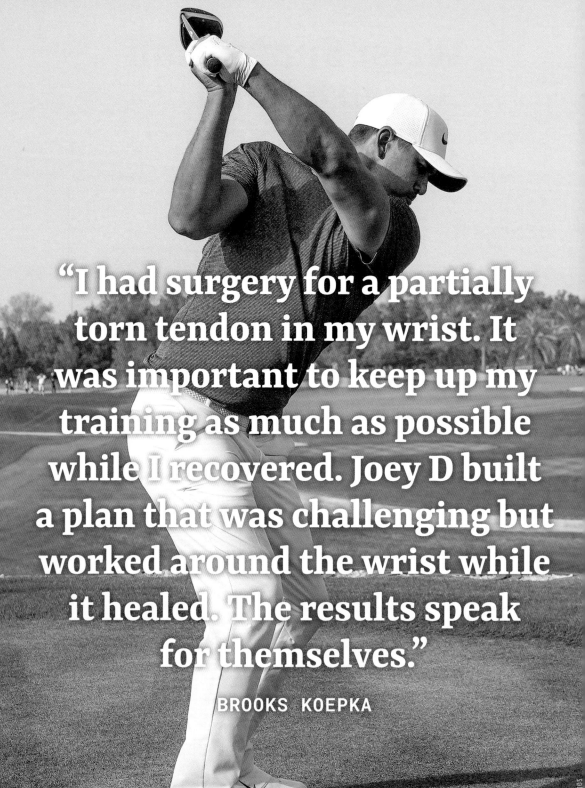

"I had surgery for a partially torn tendon in my wrist. It was important to keep up my training as much as possible while I recovered. Joey D built a plan that was challenging but worked around the wrist while it healed. The results speak for themselves."

BROOKS KOEPKA

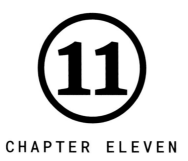

CHAPTER ELEVEN

The Wrist & Hand

There are a lot of similarities between the joints of the upper body and the joints of the lower body. The shoulders are similar to the hips, and the elbows are very much like the knees. The big difference is that while the joints of the lower body are mainly about staying connected with the ground and keeping us upright on two feet, the joints of the upper body are designed to help us deal more freely with the rest of the world. As a result, the joints of the lower body are more about stability, and the joints of the upper body are more about mobility.

We've already discussed how the anatomical differences between the ball-and-socket joints of the shoulders and the hips reflect this and how the design of the elbow lets you flip the palm of your hand over and back, while the design of the knee won't let you do the same with your foot.

This same mobility over stability theme carries over when we look at the wrists and the ankles. Because their roles and functions are different, the design of the wrists and ankles are different. The default position of the foot and ankle when standing is an incredibly stable one. The foot is flat on the ground, the ankle is flexed at 90 degrees, and you have the full weight of your body pushing straight down on the ankle joint. As far as the wrist and hand go, though, there really is no default position. Because it's designed for mobility, the range of motion at the wrist joint is far greater than that at the ankle. You can flex your wrist forward 90 degrees and you can extend it backward another roughly 90 degrees. This gives you 180 degrees of mobility forward and back. Compare that with roughly 70 degrees of combined plantarflexion and dorsiflexion at the ankle.

The wrist also flexes the hand from side to side. Put your right arm out to the side with your elbow bent at 90 degrees and your palm facing the floor with fingers pointing forward. Keeping your palm facing down, shift your hand so that your fingers are now pointing to the right. Now shift your hand so that your fingers are pointing to the left. From that same starting position, you can also flip your palm over so that it's facing up, but, as we talked about in the last chapter, this movement is actually created at the elbow.

And you can spend the next two days examining your foot and you'll never find anything as complex as the thumb. Think about all of the ways that the thumb can move. It can make contact with each of the other fingers. It can go from being parallel to the other fingers to being perpendicular to them. And from that perpendicular to the other fingers' position, it can circumduct – or rotate – in a circle in both clockwise and counterclockwise directions. The number of muscles and ligaments that allow for strength and stability for all these movements is daunting. And, again, that's just the thumb.

How complex are the wrists and hands? You actually have more bones in your pinkie finger – four – than you do in your entire arm from the shoulder down to the wrist – three. Back when we talked about the ankle, we noted that a full quarter of the bones in the human body are located in the feet. It should come as no great surprise that another quarter of them are in your hands. All those bones in your feet allow you to stay balanced under an incredible array of different situations and terrains. All those bones in your hands allow you to do – well – everything you do with your hands.

Anatomically, it's pretty easy to discuss the wrist and hand. Unlike the anatomy of the hip, which can be pretty confusing, when we talk about the wrist and hand all you have to do is look down. You can easily feel the four bones that make up each finger – the thumb only has three bones. The remaining eight bones are in the base of the hand.

In the game of golf, the hands are your body's last link to the club. We've traced the golf swing all the way from the feet up to the neck and then down the arms into the hands. Even if everything else is perfect up and down the chain, dysfunction at the wrist could still doom your golf swing. Weak wrists mean the difference between your clubhead being square to the ball at impact and your clubhead facing who-knows-where. And even if your clubhead is lucky enough to be square at impact, if

The Anatomy of the Wrist & Hand

A DETAIL OF THE JOINT, TENDONS, AND MUSCLES

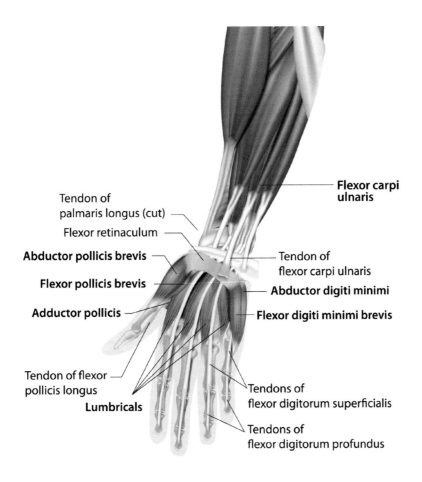

Tendon of palmaris longus (cut)

Flexor retinaculum

Abductor pollicis brevis

Flexor pollicis brevis

Adductor pollicis

Tendon of flexor pollicis longus

Lumbricals

Flexor carpi ulnaris

Tendon of flexor carpi ulnaris

Abductor digiti minimi

Flexor digiti minimi brevis

Tendons of flexor digitorum superficialis

Tendons of flexor digitorum profundus

the wrists can't hold that position confidently, there'll be some give at the moment of contact with the ball. That lack of stability at impact will cost you power and distance.

Aside from weak wrists and preexisting conditions like arthritis, the main thing you need to concern yourself about as far as the wrists and hands are concerned is injury prevention. Repetitive motions – whether it's swinging a golf club or using your computer mouse – can lead to overuse injuries. There are a lot of repetitive motions that people can get away with performing for a very long time before issues develop. Runners and swimmers can go years before experiencing overuse injuries

Get a Grip

While arthritis can affect just about any joint in the body, one of the more painful and debilitating occurrences of the disease is when it affects the hands. Instead of just feeling discomfort and tightness, when arthritis strikes the joints of the wrist and hand, it'll affect your ability to do everything from typing on a keyboard to picking up a drinking glass. And if you're a golfer, it may alter the way you've always played the game.

The most common form of arthritis in the hands and wrists is osteoarthritis. It's a wearing down of the cartilage that cushions the movement of bones at a joint. As this cartilage breaks down, there ends up being bone-on-bone contact during movement that can be incredibly painful and debilitating. The hands are vulnerable for a couple of different reasons. First, as we've mentioned, there are a whole lot of bones – and therefore joints – in the hands. The more joints, the more potential sites for arthritis to occur. Second, we use our hands for just about everything. And the more movement that joints are forced to go through – all day, every day – the greater the potential is for arthritis to show up.

Treatment for arthritis includes some commonsense things like quitting smoking, cleaning up the diet, and getting some exercise. Specific exercises that work on maintaining range of motion and strength around the joint are also recommended. Depending on the severity of the condition, you may be able to get by with just some basic lifestyle changes and some over-the-counter pain relievers. In more severe cases, prescription medications and even surgery might be necessary.

On the course, various types of hand braces have been found to ease pain for players. Another easier workaround is to switch to larger oversized grips for clubs. The larger grip requires less tension and less squeezing strength to hold.

Conveniently, the hand and wrist exercises that you should be doing anyway to help your game will also help to reduce the pain and limitations caused by arthritis. To be on the safe side, if you're currently receiving treatment for arthritis, consult your doctor before beginning any exercise program.

in the knees or shoulders. One of the reasons for this is that the muscles that operate around those joints are pretty large. Look at your hand, though. There's no room for large muscles in there. Weakness anywhere in the hand or wrist can make you a candidate for repetitive use injury.

While repetitive use injuries can happen even if every one of your swings is textbook perfect, even worse is when you're repetitively – or even occasionally – performing a less than optimal swing. The main culprit for wrist injuries on the course is chunking the ball and grabbing too much turf with your club. If you're hitting the ball cleanly, there's a minimal amount of stress at impact, because the ball doesn't weigh a whole lot and there's nothing but air preventing it from disappearing down the fairway. Your clubhead essentially makes this beautiful and stress-free trip from your backswing to your follow-through.

If your club makes contact with the ground three inches in front of your ball, though, it's a different story. The ground causes a serious and unexpected shock to the system. And this rapid deceleration is going to be felt the most profoundly in the wrists and hands. The small muscles, ligaments, and bones of the wrists and hands were designed for nimble and delicate movements like writing calligraphy and replacing the batteries in your TV remote. They weren't designed to be front seat passengers in a crash between your golf club and the ground. And the beating that your wrist and hands take every time you take a deep divot will eventually get to you. It'll not only end up affecting and altering the way you swing the club, but it will also cause you to experience wrist and hand pain in your day-to-day dealings with things like doorknobs and computer keyboards.

By strengthening the muscles that operate around the wrist, you'll be far more confident that your clubhead will be able to stay square at impact. More importantly, though, it will help prevent injury that can ruin your day both on and off the course.

Wrist Flexion/Extension

WRIST MOBILITY

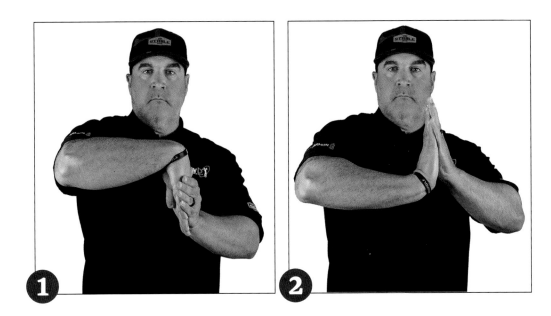

A great way to maintain proper movement at the wrist – especially if you spend a lot of your day with a keyboard and mouse.

1) Raise your right arm up in front of you with your elbow flexed at 90 degrees and the palm facing down. Your forearm should be parallel to – and directly in front of – your chest. This is the starting position.

2) With the heel of your left palm, push gently on the back of your right hand, bending your wrist as if you were trying to make your right palm touch your right forearm. You should feel a stretch on the back of your right forearm. Hold for a five-count and then return to the starting position. Now, perform the opposite movement – push on the palm of your right hand, bending your wrist back as if you were trying to get the back of your right hand to touch your forearm. You should now feel a stretch on the front of your right forearm. Hold for a five-count and return to the starting position.

Do three holds in each direction with each arm and then perform the same movements without the aid of your other hand to see if you can get the same stretch and range of motion without assistance.

Hand Extensions

HAND MOBILITY

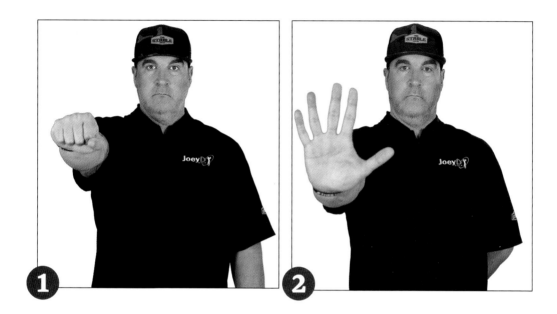

We spend most of our day with our fingers in a slightly flexed position. This is a quick and easy way to stretch through the palm and fingers. Think of it as being like yoga for your hands.

1) Make a tight fist with your right hand

2) Open your hand up and try to pull your fingers as far back as possible. You should get a stretch in your palm and into each finger. Return to the starting position to complete the rep. Do 10 extensions with each hand.

Fingertip Wall Push-Ups
WRIST/HAND STABILITY

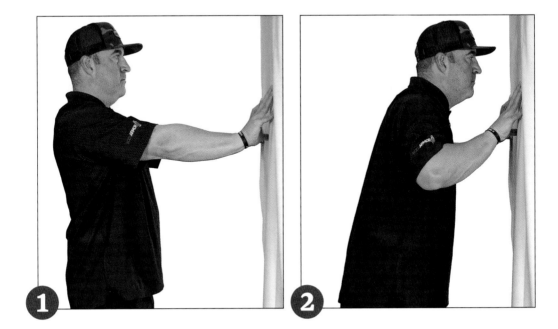

1) Stand facing a wall about two feet away from it. Place just the fingertips of both hands on the wall at chest height. Don't let your palms touch the wall. Keeping your body perfectly straight from your heels to your head, slowly lower yourself toward the wall as if you were trying to get your chest to touch it. Hold the position when your chest is about two inches from the wall. This is the starting position.

2) Keeping your body straight and just your fingertips connected to the wall, push yourself away from the wall until your arms are straight and you're almost in an upright position. Slowly lower yourself back to the starting position to complete the rep. Start by doing sets of 10 push-ups and work your way up to doing sets of 20.

Progression: Perform the same movement standing about three feet away from the wall. This time, push off the wall so explosively that your fingertips come off the wall. Try to push yourself back onto your heels. Fall forward back toward the wall and – using just your fingertips – gently decelerate your body back to the starting position without letting your chest (or your face!) touch the wall. Again, start with sets of 10 and work your way up to sets of 20.

Wrist Curls

FOREARM STRENGTH AT THE WRIST

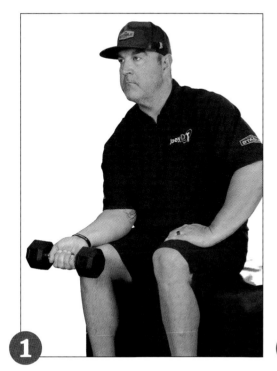

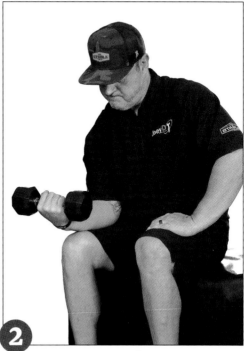

1) Sit comfortably with feet about hip-width apart. Holding a light dumbbell in your right hand, rest your forearm on your right thigh with your palm facing up. Your wrist and hand should be hanging over your thigh, past your knee. Let the weight roll down your hand until you're holding it in your fingertips. This is the starting position.

2) Begin the movement by lifting the weight up by curling the fingers into a fist. This will target the muscles in the palm and fingers. Keeping your forearm against your thigh, continue the movement by raising your fist up by bending at the wrist. This will target the muscles in the forearm that flex the wrist. Hold this position for a moment and then slowly lower the weight back to the starting position to complete the rep. Shoot for sets of 20 on both the right and left side.

Reverse Wrist Curls
FOREARM STRENGTH AT THE WRIST

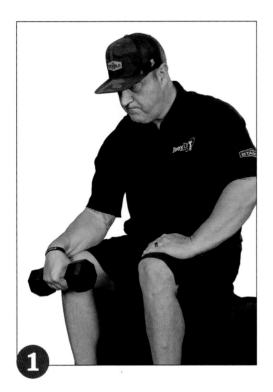
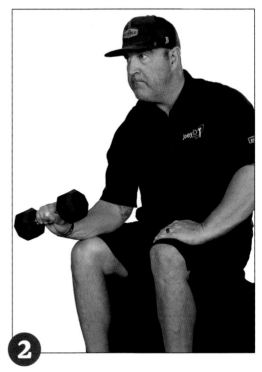

1) To work the muscles that extend the wrist backward, assume the same starting position as the previous movement, but with your palm facing down and your hand already in a fist. With the weight in your hand, your wrist should be bent to almost 90 degrees in this position. You may want to go with an even lighter weight than in the last exercise.

2) Keeping your forearm tight against your thigh, lift the weight by pulling your fist up and back. Hold the position for a beat and then slowly return to the starting position to complete the rep. The key is to keep your forearm from moving, which is what it's going to want to do. Do sets of 20 reps on each side. If you haven't done any wrist or forearm exercises before, you will feel these pretty quickly.

Lateral Wrist Raises

FOREARM STRENGTH AT THE WRIST

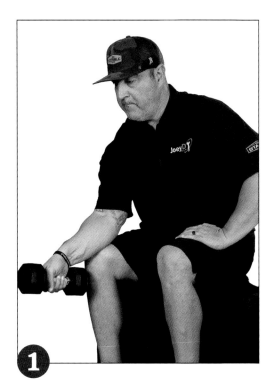

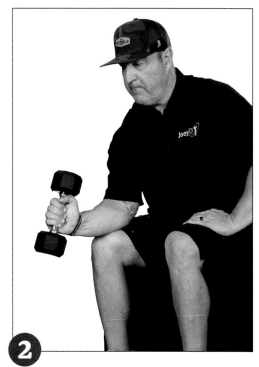

1) To work the muscles that move the hand to the left and right, use the same setup position as on the previous page, but with the palm of your right hand facing to the left. The dumbbell will almost be in a vertical position. Keeping your forearm tight against your thigh, tilt the dumbbell forward as if it were a microphone and you were interviewing someone sitting directly in front of you. This is the starting position.

2) Without moving the forearm, pull the dumbbell backward until it's angled toward you. (If you want to stick to the microphone analogy, it now should be aimed at you.) Hold this position for a second and then slowly return to the starting position. Shoot for sets of 20 reps on each side.

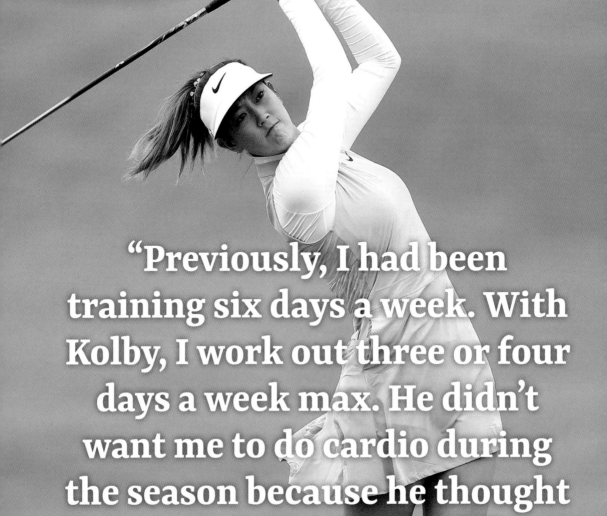

"Previously, I had been training six days a week. With Kolby, I work out three or four days a week max. He didn't want me to do cardio during the season because he thought it would be too much."

MICHELLE WIE

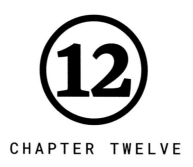

CHAPTER TWELVE

The Workout

Congratulations! You've just read through a whole lot of theory and science and now you're about to embark on some serious application and experience some serious progress. These are the same exercises and this is the same workout program used by the best golfers in the world.

In. The. World.

There are no shortcuts and there are no "secrets" to playing better. There is only work and dedication. This is the blueprint. This is the process. Trust the process, work hard, and you'll be amazed at how well you'll soon be playing. Trust, train, and win. The best golfers on the planet prepare their bodies to play using this same process. And the season favors the prepared!

Trust. Train. Win.

Now you know the theories behind our Species-Specific-Before-Sports-Specific philosophy as well as the anatomy and design of the major joints of the body and how they need to function properly in the golf swing. (You also now know how dysfunction at any of the major joints will negatively affect your swing.)

It's time to put the workouts and your workout schedule together. This is one of the more unique workout programs that you may ever do. And it's not just different for the sake of being different; it's different because there's over 50 years of combined strength, conditioning, and biomechanics experience behind it. There's no guesswork or wasted movement in these workouts. Everything you do will be geared toward making you function much better as a human and play much better as a golfer.

If you've ever been on an exercise program, the thing that's probably been the toughest to deal with is the repetition of doing the same movements over and over again. This can be soul-crushing and self-defeating on a couple of different levels. First of all, it can be deathly boring. If you're always doing the same chest presses and the same leg extensions at exactly the same points in your workout, the whole experience can make you feel like a laboratory rat simply going through the motions. Once this has happened, you've checked out emotionally and you honestly would rather be doing anything else in the world other than those same chest presses and leg extensions.

"I'll tell Kolby, 'Man, I don't want a real hard workout' or 'I want a real hard workout,' but he'll know when he can go hard. If it's five workouts, a few weeks in a row, bring on the heat. But if it's the first week in, you're trying to just get going." – **Harold Varner III**

On the physiological front, doing the same movements over and over again is a surefire way to hit a plateau and stop improving. Your body has learned how to adapt to these movements. Early on, these movements and exercises might have been challenging, but your body has figured them out and is no longer challenged by them. It would be like learning to read by spending two hours every week rereading and reviewing the words "cat" and "dog." At some point, you need to move on and challenge yourself with words like "catapult" and "dogmatic."

(And if you were already feeling like a laboratory rat just going through the motions, the fact that you're no longer seeing any progress will make you feel that you're a lab rat in the control group designed for failure.)

This is what we talked about when we were discussing the importance of neuromuscular training. The key isn't just to move your body (or a weight) from point A to point B; the key to constant improvement is to continually tweak what happens between point A and point B. This forces continual adaptations to occur and as these adaptations occur, so do your improvements in strength, balance, coordination, and agility.

We took the 40-plus different mobility, stability, and strength moves in the program and put them together in such a way that you'll easily be able to work out three times a week for an entire month without repeating the same workout twice. And with all of the progressions of the exercises we've included, this may feel like the least "routine" exercise program you've ever been on. Not only will this keep the workouts fresh and exciting for you, it'll challenge and stimulate your neuromuscular system unlike any other workout you've ever done.

But while your skeletal system, muscular system, and nervous system will find the workouts incredibly complex and challenging, we want to keep things pretty simple for you when it comes to putting things together. You don't need to join a gym to do this program and you don't need to have or to buy a ton of expensive equipment. Other than a golf club and golf ball (which we're pretty sure you have), the only other equipment required is light-, medium-, and heavy-resistance bands, one medium resistance looped band, a light (5-8 pound) pair of dumbbells, a heavier (10-15 pound) pair of dumbbells, inexpensive furniture sliders, and a stability ball. That's probably less than a $150 investment in your body and your game.

Oh, and we also want you to get a notebook. Most exercise programs are obsessed with weight; your success or failure on any given day is how heavy you lifted. If you lifted more than you did last week, that must mean you're improving, and if you didn't lift as much, that must mean you're slipping. If you take a look at the list of equipment you'll need for the program, you'll realize that there are no heavy weights. No stacks of 45-pound plates to whip around and no 60-pound dumbbells to play with. We did this on purpose.

It's not the quantity of weight that you move, it's the quality of the way that you move it that counts. The gyms of America are full of guys who can squat 315 or 405 pounds incorrectly. There's weakness at the ankles and knees and no stability at the hips or back. Yes, technically, it may meet the definition of a squat, but it's really a series of dysfunctional movements with injury waiting to jump in at any point. If we're choosing sides for just about any sport that people play, all day long we're going for the person who can squat 225 – or 135 – with proper form.

This is not a "no pain, no gain" workout. Sure, there's a time to go heavy and see just how much weight you can move, but this is about optimizing your body to play golf, not about optimizing your body to be an NFL defensive lineman. Knowing which exercises will move you closer to your goal – and knowing which exercises to avoid –

is vital. And overtraining is not a "badge of honor," but a surefire way to derail you from reaching your goal.

We get success with our players not by focusing on basic stats like the amount of weight they're lifting; we get results by focusing on how stable, powerful, and efficient their movements are. (Don't get us wrong – you'll be dealing with plenty of heavy resistance during these workouts, and there will be days when you may wake up sore. Your next-day soreness, though, is by no means any measure of "success.")

The notebook is going to be your way to keep track of your progress. We want you to write down how the different exercises felt. Was maintaining your balance on a particular exercise easier than it was the last time you did it? Are you finding more mobility at the ankles or neck than you did a month ago? Has an exercise become more fluid and stable over the course of the program? These are the real signs of improvement or progress.

You don't have to write a lot – a few lines or words is all. We'd rather have you concentrating on your form and movement than your writing skills, but you'd be amazed at how something as simple as putting words on paper cements it in time and lets you truly see how much your body – and your awareness of your body – is changing.

At the end of this chapter, we've included a month's worth of workouts. The players we work with are busy people and so are you. We don't need you working out every day. We've structured the program into three workouts per week, each lasting roughly half an hour. This might not seem like a lot, but because the workouts are laser-focused on improving what we know are the key components to proper function, there's no wasted movement and, as a result, no wasted time.

> *"It's like less is more. The workouts are so specific to you and to golf. I thought you had to work out multiple hours every day. I've felt the best I ever have just by working out three or four times a week versus every day. I don't think I've ever not felt good after a workout. Whereas before, I would just feel shot."*
> – Jaye Marie Green

For each workout, we want you to first review each of the exercises listed to make sure that you know exactly what to do and that you have the right equipment handy. You may also want to review your notes about the last time you did the same exercises to see if there are certain aspects of the moves that you particularly want to focus on. After that, spend about five minutes getting your body warm and your mind prepped. You can use a treadmill, elliptical, or stationary bike if you have one or simply jog in place, shadow box, or jump rope. Use this warm-up time to get yourself mentally ready for your workout. Because the workout is designed to challenge you on multiple levels, it's important to connect your brain to your body as much as possible.

Because the structure and complexity of each joint is different, some workouts may skew more toward mobility or stability moves as opposed to strength moves. In any case, we want you to go through all of the mobility exercises first, then hit the stability movements, and then – finally – the strength moves. For each of the groupings – mobility, stability, and strength – cycle three times through the movements listed to keep your nervous system continually engaged.

Between sets is when you'd break out your notebook to write down any thoughts you had about a particular exercise.

Continue to cycle through the workouts after you've completed the first month. As far as the variations and progressions of the exercises go, feel free to swap in the exercise variations whenever you want. For the progressions, wait until you can comfortably and fluidly perform an exercise before moving on to its next progression. That said, we'd like you to finish at least two complete cycles of the workout before adding any progressions.

Okay, you've just done a ton of reading, it's time to get to work!

Week One

WORKOUT 1

EXERCISE	PURPOSE	SETS	REPS	PAGE
Cat/Cow Stretch	Spinal Mobility	3	10	106
Golf Ball Foot Hurdles	Ankle & Foot Mobility	3	10	54
Follow-Through with Bands	Spinal Mobility	3	10	108
Single-Leg Standing Balance	Ankle Stability	3	3	56
Standing Anti-Rotation with Bands	Spinal Stability	3	4	110
Standing Calf Raise	Calf Strength at the Ankle	3	30	58
Standing Row with Bands	Back Strength at the Spine	3	10	112
Toe Raises with Looped Band	Anterior Strength at the Ankle	3	10	59
Single Arm Row on One Foot	Back Strength at the Spine	3	10	114

WORKOUT 2

EXERCISE	PURPOSE	SETS	REPS	PAGE
Standing Hip Opener	Hip Mobility	3	10	88
Wrist Flexion/Extension	Wrist Mobility	3	3	172
Hand Extensions	Hand Mobility	3	10	173
Hip Tilt with Stability Ball	Hip Mobility	3	10	86
Lateral Movement with Looped Band	Hip Stability	3	5	89
Fingertip Wall Push-Ups	Wrist/Hand Stability	3	20	174
Wrist Curls	Forearm Strength at the Wrist	3	20	175
Hip Bridges	Glute Strength at the Hips	3	25	92
Reverse Wrist Curls	Forearm Strength at the Wrist	3	20	176
Lateral Wrist Raises	Forearm Strength at the Wrist	3	20	177

WORKOUT 3

EXERCISE	PURPOSE	SETS	REPS	PAGE
Internal Rotation with Band	Shoulder Mobility	3	10	142
External Rotation with Band	Shoulder Mobility	3	10	144
Biceps Stretch	Elbow Mobility	3	3	156
Forearm Slides	Shoulder Stability	3	10	140
Straight Arm Planks	Elbow Stability	3	3	158
Wrist Pronation with Band	Forearm Strength at the Elbow	3	10	164
Wrist Supination with Band	Forearm Strength at the Elbow	3	10	165
Shoulder Blade Retraction with Bands	Back Strength at the Shoulder	3	10	148
Triceps Extensions with Bands	Triceps Strength at the Elbow	3	10	160
Single-Arm Flies with Band	Chest Strength at the Shoulder	3	10	146

Week Two

EXERCISE	PURPOSE	SETS	REPS	PAGE
Omnidirectional Movement	Neck Mobility	3	5	124
Romanian Deadlift	Knee Mobility/Hamstring Strength	3	10	70
Rotation with Eyes on the Ball	Neck Stability	3	10	128
Lunges with Rotation	Knee Stability	3	10	72
Hamstring Curls	Hamstring Strength at the Knees	3	20	76
Manual Resistance (five-count hold)	Neck Strength	3	1	130
Split Lunge	Quadriceps Strength at Knee	3	20	74

WORKOUT 2

EXERCISE	PURPOSE	SETS	REPS	PAGE
Cat/Cow Stretch	Spinal Mobility	3	10	106
Follow-Through with Bands	Spinal Mobility	3	10	108
Wrist Flexion/Extension	Wrist Mobility	3	3	172
Hand Extensions	Hand Mobility	3	10	173
Standing Anti-Rotation with Bands	Spinal Stability	3	4	110
Fingertip Wall Push-Ups	Wrist/Hand Stability	3	20	174
Standing Row with Bands	Back Strength at the Spine	3	10	112
Wrist Curls	Forearm Strength at the Wrist	3	20	175
Reverse Wrist Curls	Forearm Strength at the Wrist	3	20	176
Lateral Wrist Raises	Forearm Strength at the Wrist	3	20	177
Single Arm Row on One Foot	Back Strength at the Spine	3	10	114

WORKOUT 3

EXERCISE	PURPOSE	SETS	REPS	PAGE
Standing Hip Opener	Hip Mobility	3	10	88
Hip Tilt with Stability Ball	Hip Mobility	3	10	86
Biceps Stretch	Elbow Mobility	3	10	156
Straight Arm Planks	Elbow Stability	3	10	158
Lateral Movement with Looped Band	Hip Stability	3	5	89
Triceps Extensions with Bands	Triceps Strength at the Elbow	3	10	160
Wrist Pronation with Band	Forearm Strength at the Elbow	3	10	164
Wrist Supination with Band	Forearm Strength at the Elbow	3	10	165
Hip Bridges	Glute Strength at the Hips	3	25	92

Week Three

WORKOUT 1

EXERCISE	PURPOSE	SETS	REPS	PAGE
Internal Rotation with Band	Shoulder Mobility	3	10	142
External Rotation with Band	Shoulder Mobility	3	10	144
Omnidirectional Movement	Neck Mobility	3	5	124
Forearm Slides	Shoulder Stability	3	10	140
Rotation with Eyes on the Ball	Neck Stability	3	10	128
Shoulder Blade Retraction with Bands	Back Strength at the Shoulder	3	10	148
Single-Arm Flies with Band	Chest Strength at the Shoulder	3	10	146
Manual Resistance (five-count hold)	Neck Strength	3	1	130

WORKOUT 2

EXERCISE	PURPOSE	SETS	REPS	PAGE
Golf Ball Foot Hurdles	Ankle & Foot Mobility	3	10	54
Romanian Deadlift	Knee Mobility/Hamstring Strength	3	10	70
Single-Leg Standing Balance	Ankle Stability	3	3	56
Lunges with Rotation	Knee Stability	3	10	72
Toe Raises with Looped Band	Anterior Strength at the Ankle	3	10	59
Hamstring Curls	Hamstring Strength at the Knees	3	20	76
Split Lunge	Quadriceps Strength at the Knee	3	20	74
Standing Calf Raise	Calf Strength at the Ankle	3	30	58

WORKOUT 3

EXERCISE	PURPOSE	SETS	REPS	PAGE
Cat/Cow Stretch	Spinal Mobility	3	10	106
Biceps Stretch	Elbow Mobility	3	3	156
Follow-Through with Bands	Spinal Mobility	3	10	108
Standing Anti-Rotation with Bands	Spinal Stability	3	4	110
Straight Arm Planks	Elbow Stability	3	3	158
Standing Row with Bands	Back Strength at the Spine	3	10	112
Wrist Pronation with Band	Forearm Strength at the Elbow	3	10	164
Wrist Supination with Band	Forearm Strength at the Elbow	3	10	165
Single Arm Row on One Foot	Back Strength at the Spine	3	10	114
Triceps Extensions with Bands	Triceps Strength at the Elbow	3	10	160

Week Four

WORKOUT 1

EXERCISE	PURPOSE	SETS	REPS	PAGE
Standing Hip Opener	Hip Mobility	3	10	88
Hip Tilt with Stability Ball	Hip Mobility	3	10	86
Omnidirectional Movement	Neck Mobility	3	5	124
Lateral Movement with Looped Band	Hip Stability	3	5	89
Rotation with Eyes on the Ball	Neck Stability	3	10	128
Hip Bridges	Glute Strength at the Hips	3	25	92
Manual Resistance (five-count hold)	Neck Strength	3	1	130

WORKOUT 2

EXERCISE	PURPOSE	SETS	REPS	PAGE
Internal Rotation with Band	Shoulder Mobility	3	10	142
External Rotation with Band	Shoulder Mobility	3	10	144
Golf Ball Foot Hurdles	Ankle & Foot Mobility	3	10	54
Forearm Slides	Shoulder Stability	3	10	140
Single-Leg Standing Balance	Ankle Stability	3	3	56
Toe Raises with Looped Band	Anterior Strength at the Ankle	3	10	59
Shoulder Blade Retraction with Bands	Back Strength at the Shoulder	3	10	148
Standing Calf Raise	Calf Strength at the Ankle	3	30	58
Single-Arm Flies with Band	Chest Strength at the Shoulder	3	10	146

WORKOUT 3

EXERCISE	PURPOSE	SETS	REPS	PAGE
Romanian Deadlift	Knee Mobility/Hamstring Strength	3	10	70
Wrist Flexion/Extension	Wrist Mobility	3	3	172
Hand Extensions	Hand Mobility	3	10	173
Lunges with Rotation	Knee Stability	3	10	72
Fingertip Wall Push-Ups	Wrist/Hand Stability	3	20	174
Hamstring Curls	Hamstring Strength at the Knees	3	20	76
Wrist Curls	Forearm Strength at the Wrist	3	20	175
Reverse Wrist Curls	Forearm Strength at the Wrist	3	20	176
Lateral Wrist Raises	Forearm Strength at the Wrist	3	20	177
Split Lunge	Quadriceps Strength at the Knee	3	20	74

For example, here's how you'd do your first workout:

Five-minute warm-up and mental prep

Mobility:
Cat/Cow Stretch

Golf Ball Foot Hurdles

Follow-Through with Bands

Cat/Cow Stretch

Golf Ball Foot Hurdles

Follow-Through with Bands

Cat/Cow Stretch

Golf Ball Foot Hurdles

Follow-Through with Bands

Stability:
Single-Leg Standing Balance

Standing Anti-Rotation with Bands

Single-Leg Standing Balance

Standing Anti-Rotation with Bands

Single-Leg Standing Balance

Standing Anti-Rotation with Bands

Strength:
Standing Calf Raise

Standing Row with Bands

Toe Raises with Looped Band

Single Arm Row on One Foot

Standing Calf Raise

Standing Row with Bands

Toe Raises with Looped Band

Single Arm Row on One Foot

Standing Calf Raise

Standing Row with Bands

Toe Raises with Looped Band

Single Arm Row on One Foot

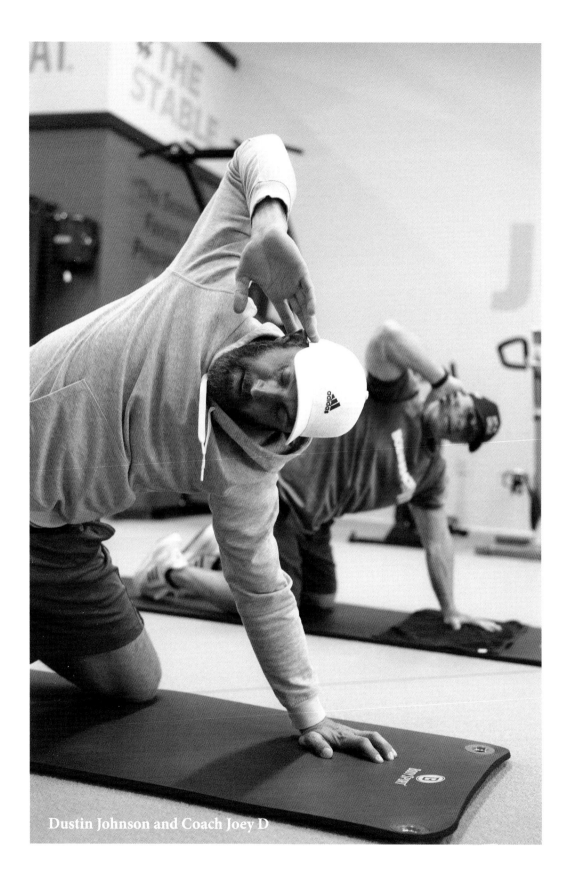

Dustin Johnson and Coach Joey D

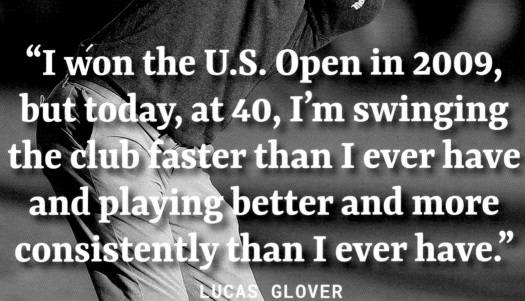

"I won the U.S. Open in 2009, but today, at 40, I'm swinging the club faster than I ever have and playing better and more consistently than I ever have."

LUCAS GLOVER

CHAPTER THIRTEEN

On the Course

You now know exactly what to do off the course to prepare your body to not only function more properly as a human, but also to function more properly as a golfer. We're confident that after reading the science behind what we do here at the Joey D Golf Sports Training Center, you now understand at a very deep level everything that has to happen – from your toes all the way to your fingers – to swing a golf club properly. And we're confident that the deeper you get into this workout program, the easier, stronger, and more stable your own swing will begin to feel.

But just because you've trained your body to swing the club better than you've ever thought possible, it doesn't mean you can just roll out of bed at 7:00, arrive at the course at 7:55, and shoot lights-out golf at 8:00. You can't. No one can.

You also can't sit at your desk all day, sit for another hour while you drive to the course, pull your clubs out of your trunk at 5:55 and expect to shoot lights-out golf at 6:00. You can't. No one can.

Of course, you can try to do either of those things – and we're sure you've attempted both of them more times than you'd like to admit. You just won't play all that well. In a best-case scenario, you'll spend the first three holes "loosening up" and getting a feel for your game. And by the time you've discovered your swing, your score could be well north of par. In a worst-case scenario, your body just isn't ready to corkscrew itself into your backswing and you'll end up tweaking any number of the dozens of muscles we've mentioned in this book. Pros, of course, don't have the luxury of loosening up while they play. A bad score on any hole – whether it's the first hole on Thursday morning or the last hole on Sunday afternoon – can negatively affect the leaderboard and their bank account.

"From the outside, golf doesn't look like an endurance sport. You don't run. You don't jump. There's explosiveness in the swing, but people don't think about the endurance part. It's a whole week of mentally draining competition. And you do it week after week after week. Feeling physically fit for me was very important. And that also helped me with the mental side of the game as well."
– **Beatriz Recari**

Most pros arrive at the course hours before their actual tee time. Hours. If you're wondering why you don't see a lot of late-night scandals involving pro golfers, it's because they're usually in bed by 8:00.

We don't expect you to be at the course at 5:00 in the morning for a 7:00 tee time, but we do want you to put as much thought and effort into your pre-round preparation as you've put into everything else we've talked about so far.

If you can be at the course 30 to 45 minutes before you're supposed to play, you'll have ample time to prep your body physically to play your best golf from your opening drive. And being able to get into a dedicated warm-up routine will also let you prep for your round mentally. You'll have the time to distance yourself from worries about work, family, money, and whatever else can get lodged in your subconscious and keep you from focusing on your game. Heading onto the first tee with the proper mental attitude and a body that's been primed to play will give you an immediate advantage over everyone else you're teeing off against. Let them spend the first three holes getting a feel for their game while you go chasing birdies from the outset.

"Kolby improves everybody. Even if your body is where you want it to be, with all the travel that we do and all the swinging that we do, at some point in time, something's going to give. There's been a couple of times when we've been at tournaments and I'm thinking: 'Man, I am so glad that you're here.' When he's there, my body is 100 percent ready to go, every time." – **Andrew Loupe**

Just like everything else in this book, this pre-round warm-up isn't guesswork. It's not the same three-minute series of half-hearted stretches that you see every other golfer do in the parking lot before they play. It's designed to mobilize your body,

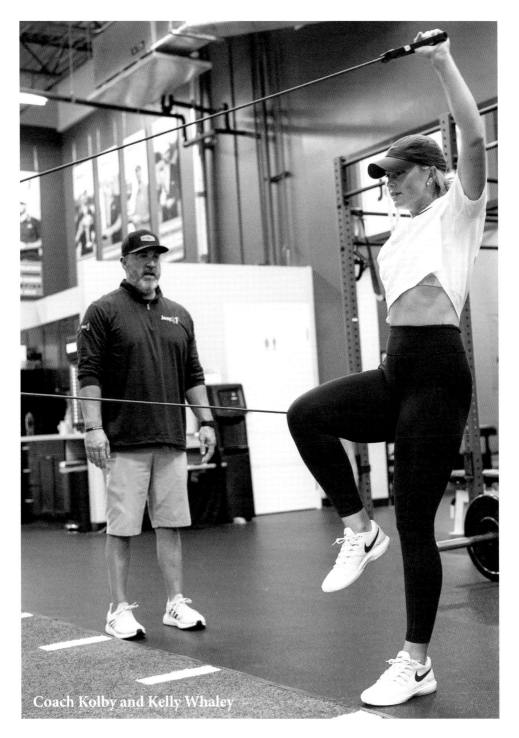

Coach Kolby and Kelly Whaley

awaken your nervous system, and engage the muscles required for swinging the club properly. And just as we did when we began discussing the joints of the body, we're going to prep you to play by starting from the ground and moving up. Find a grassy area where you have some space to move and you'll be amazed at how ready to play you'll feel after doing these six warm-up movements.

Pendulum Swing with Leg Supported by Club

ON-COURSE WARM-UP

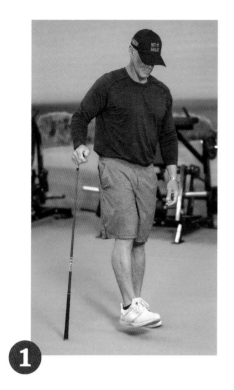

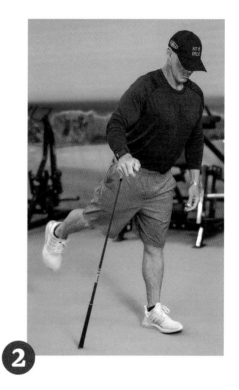

1) To get your hip flexors and quads on the front of your body and your lower back, glutes, and hamstrings on the back of your body ready for action, grab a long iron or a driver in your right hand and plant the grip end in the ground directly to your right.

2) Ground your left foot firmly on the grass and begin to swing your right leg forward and back. Try to keep your knee from bending, but you might find that difficult to do initially. (On the plus side, over time, you'll notice that it becomes easier and easier to keep your leg straight during this stretch. This is some nice proof of progress!)

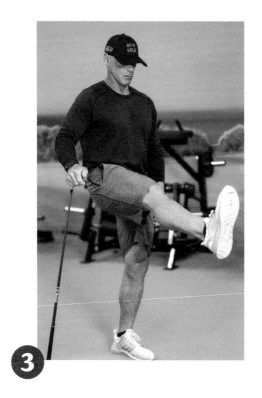

3) Start slowly. As things start to get looser, you'll find your leg being able to go a little bit higher both forward and back. There'll be a tendency to want to rock your upper body back and forth to help with the movement, but try to keep your upper body quiet and tall. You want to feel a stretch in your hips, but you don't want to feel a strain. You're getting ready to play golf, not blast 60-yard punts for the Miami Dolphins.

Do 20 forward-and-back swings with the right leg and then switch the club to your left hand and do 20 pendulum swings with the left leg.

Deadlift with Club

ON-COURSE WARM-UP

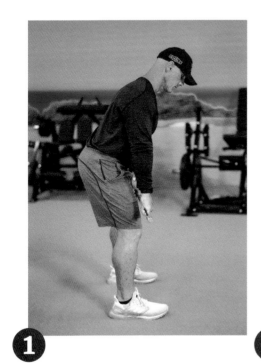

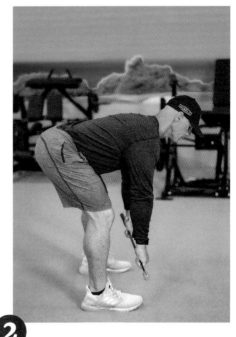

This one is going to hit a lot of notes, but that makes sense since it's based on a deadlift, which is one of the best full-body strength moves out there. It'll prep your hips for proper hinging at address. It'll continue to stretch the hamstrings, glutes, and lower back. And it'll even start to open up the chest and shoulders.

1) Assume an address position with proper golf posture while holding a club horizontally across your upper thighs with straight arms. This is the starting position.

2) Keeping your back straight and hinging only at the hips, lower your upper body and slide the club along your thighs until it's just below knee level. Hold for a second to feel the stretch in your hamstrings and lower back and then, keeping the club against your body, stand straight up and pull your shoulders back to get a stretch across your chest. Drop back into the starting position and repeat the movement trying to go a little lower with your upper back, so that the club is now lower on your shins. With each rep, try to go a little lower with the club until you're reaching your ankles.

The key is to keep the back straight and hinge properly at the hips without rounding the lower or upper back. Don't rush things. Go only as deep as you can with proper form. Shoot for 15 reps.

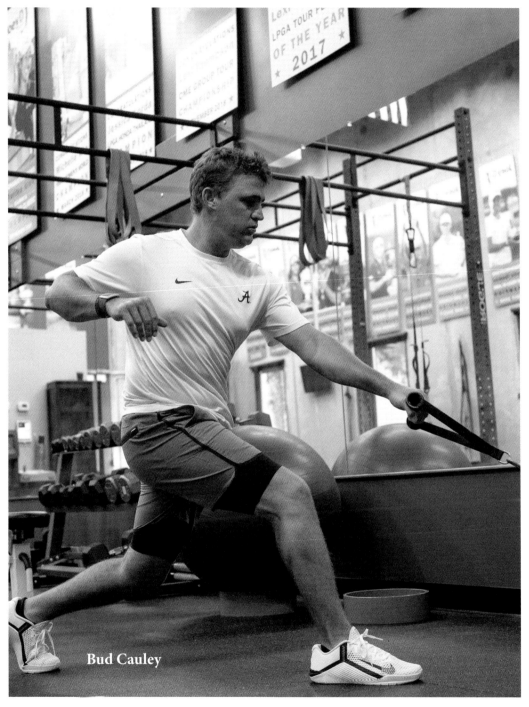

Bud Cauley

Reverse Lunge with Twist

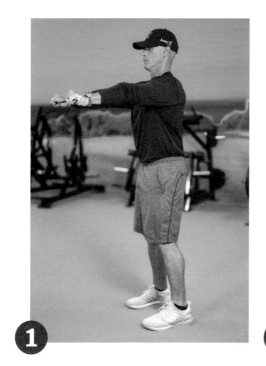
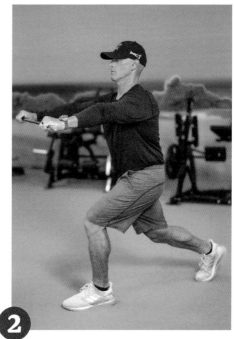

1) This is going to be similar to the Lunges with Rotation exercise from the Knee chapter, but with one major difference. Stand with your feet shoulder-width apart holding a club out in front of you horizontally at shoulder height. Your hands should be slightly wider than shoulder-width apart. This is the starting position.

2) Now, instead of taking a deep step forward into a lunge position as you did in the earlier exercise, you're going to take a big step back with your right leg until you're in a left-leg-forward lunge position. So, before you're even going to get a chance to feel the nice stretch in your right hip, you're going to have to deal with some interesting balance issues. First, stepping backward so deeply and trying to stabilize yourself is no easy task. In addition, since you're doing this on grass and not on a solid workout floor, you're also going to be dealing with unstable surfaces. Put these two things together and you've got your nervous system firing on all cylinders.

3) In the lunge position, your left knee should be directly over your left heel and your left knee should be bent to around 90 degrees. Once you've stabilized yourself, and

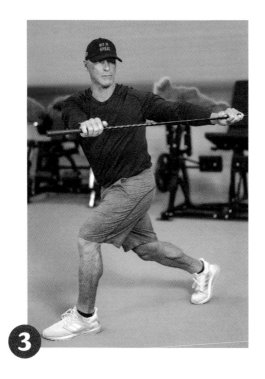

it might take longer than you think, slowly rotate your upper body toward the left, while maintaining a very upright posture and keeping the club extended out in front of you at shoulder height. Make sure to turn your head as you turn your upper body. This will not only let you rotate a little deeper, but because it's going to force you to move your eyes from a stable focal point, it'll also challenge your balance more. Hold this position for a second and then return to a forward-facing lunge position. Once again, find your balance and then rotate your upper body to the right – or away from your lead leg. Hold this position for a second and then return to the forward-facing lunge position. Finally, step your right leg forward to return to the starting position and to complete the rep.

In addition to prepping your system for whatever balance, stability, and footing issues the course is going to throw at you, you're also opening up the hips and getting in some good spinal rotation. Do 10 reps, alternating between stepping back with the right leg and stepping back with the left leg.

Three Step Squat / Chest Opener with Club

ON-COURSE WARM-UP

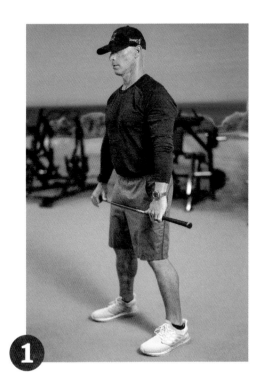
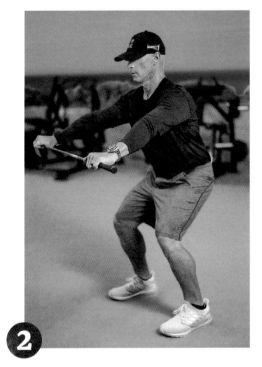

1) To keep your round-prep going and to get your upper body and lower body in sync with each other, stand with your feet slightly wider than shoulder-width apart while holding a club horizontally across your hips with straight arms. This is the starting position.

2) Slowly drop your hips by bending your knees, while at the same time raise the club in front of you with both arms. As you lower yourself, make sure you are hinging properly at the hips and not rounding your lower back. Try to keep your arms straight and not bend at the elbow. Feel your glutes and quads engage and a slight stretch into your chest and shoulders and then return to the starting position.

For the first five reps, only drop the hips slightly (while making sure your knees stay aligned over your heels) and raise the club only to about neck height.

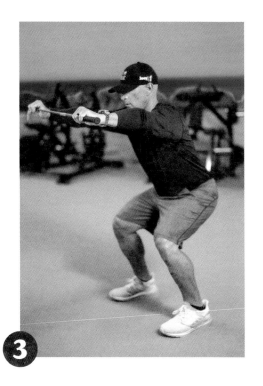
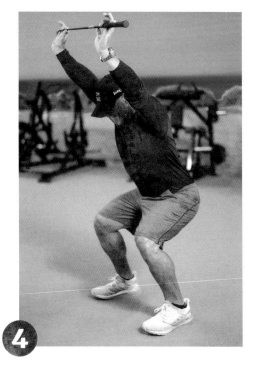

3) For the next five, try to drop the hips a little bit deeper while maintaining good form and try to get the club to forehead height with straight arms. For the final five, drop as low as you can with your hips with proper alignment while raising the club as high as you can with your arms fully extended. The goal is to get your knees to 90 degrees and the club over your head. It probably won't happen on day one, but when it does, you'll once again have some satisfying proof of progress.

4) See how smoothly you can transfer from the first five to the second five to the third five as you go through this 15-rep set.

Thoracic Opener

ON-COURSE WARM-UP

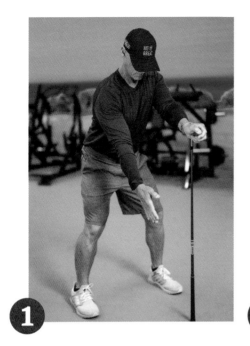 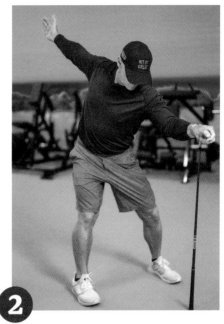

1) To keep the chest and shoulders open while loosening through the thoracic spine, assume an address position. Holding a long iron or driver in your left hand, extend your left arm fully and plant the grip end in the ground. The club should be vertical and your two feet and the grip end of the club should form a triangle on the ground. Your right arm should be straight and extended slightly forward and down – as it would be at address. This is the starting position.

2) Keeping your right arm straight and maintaining your spine angle, sweep your arm back until your fingers are pointing at the sky. Ideally, you want this movement to occur smoothly in your swing plane. Feel a stretch across your chest and into your shoulders and return to the starting position while continuing to keep your right arm straight.

Do 10 reps with your right arm and then 10 reps with your left arm. You may notice a slight – or not so slight – difference in your ability to turn on one side versus the other. This is normal. The goal, though, is to reduce this asymmetry over time.

Single-Leg Rotation

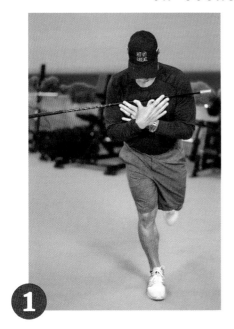 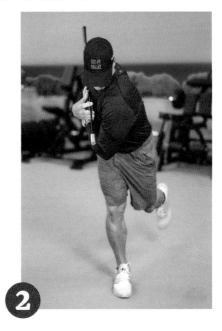

Finally, we're going to tie everything together with a move that checks a lot of boxes. This one will work on rotation around the hips and spine, engage the stabilizers in the legs and the postural muscles in the back, and challenge your balance.

1) Assume a narrow-stanced setup position while holding a club horizontally across your chest with crossed arms. Knees should be slightly bent and you should be hinged properly at the hips. This will allow you to maintain your golf posture without rounding your back. Bend your left knee to raise your left foot slightly off the floor in back of you. This is the starting position.

2) Keeping your head in a fixed position and your eyes on where your ball would be, rotate your upper body to the right, into what would be your backswing (for righties). Try to keep your chest up and avoid rounding your upper back. Hold your backswing for a moment and then slowly rotate back to the starting position. Go slow. This is a tough one. The goal is to be able to perform a controlled movement despite the instability. If balance is an issue, start with a more limited backswing and gradually add more rotation over time. The good news is that when this move feels comfortable, you're definitely ready to play your round. Do 10 rotations to the right and then switch feet and do 10 rotations to the left.

Science and the Golf Club

Because you've read this far, you're obviously not intimidated by the science behind the game. As you can probably tell, we're not of the "grip it and rip it" school of thought. We've meticulously broken down the human body, joint-by-joint, to show you how every part of this amazing machine has its own role in the golf swing and how dysfunction at even one joint can derail an otherwise beautiful golf swing.

But the swing doesn't end at your fingertips. Your body doesn't hit the ball. Your body swings the club that hits the ball. You could have followed to the letter everything we've had you do in this book, but if the clubs you're playing with aren't in tune with your body and your swing, you won't be hitting things as optimally as you could be. We're not going to get overly analytical about golf club physics, because, well, that would mean we'd have to write a whole other book, but we did want to briefly mention some of the science behind using the correct clubs.

The height of the average adult American male is around 5'9" and it's about 5'4" for the average adult female. If you're taller or shorter than these averages, then any stock club that you're playing with is going to force you into some sort of compensation without you even realizing it. If you're a taller person, you're going to be playing with clubs that are too short for you and as a result, you'll need to somehow get lower at your address to be in a position to hit the ball. Now, you're either needing more knee bend or a deeper hinge at the hips. If you can't lower yourself in these ways, you're going to end up rounding your back to be in a position to hit the ball. And even if you've just skimmed the pages of this book up until now, you would have already seen no shortage of warnings about the dangers of playing with a rounded back. Everything from lack of power and accuracy to potential chronic back pain can result from playing in a stooped over position.

If you're shorter than average, then you're going to be playing with clubs that are too long for you. You'll need to set up farther away from the ball or you're going to have to stand up too tall at address. Both of these will alter your swing plane and affect the way the clubface strikes the ball and that's going to affect accuracy.

Odds are, though, unless you're a junior player, your height isn't going to dramatically change over time. But, if your body and swing have been changing due to the workouts in this book, you may want to make sure the flex of your shafts is appropriate for your new level of play.

Shaft flex is the amount the shaft will bend during your swing. In general, a softer, more flexible shaft is a little lighter and more forgiving, helping players with less speed and power gain a bit more launch – thus more carry distance – than a stiffer shaft. A stiffer shaft will tend to launch a lower ball flight, but unless you can generate decent speed and power, you're going to sacrifice carry and overall distance.

Unfortunately, shaft flex is broken down into a handful of nonstandardized ratings that might influence your purchasing decisions in a counterproductive way and prevent you from playing with shafts that are right for you. Forced to choose between X (extra stiff), S (stiff), R (regular), A (senior), and L (ladies), many players might assume that since they're neither older nor a female, they should be playing a regular shaft. And that might be the wrong decision for their body and their swing. There are some very rough guidelines designed to tell you what shaft you should be using, but these are primarily based on driving distance and not on the tempo, timing, and speed of your swing.

Of course, all of this can change based on the weight of the clubhead. (We told you golf club physics was a whole other book!) Essentially, though, this is why we have our own club fitters – ClubCraft – on premises at the Joey D Golf Sports Training Center. The club is the last link between the body and the ball. And just as we want to create a seamless transfer of energy and power from the ankles up through the knees and hips, we also want that same seamless transfer down from the shoulders through the elbows and wrists and then through the club to the ball.

Not everyone has the money to get custom fit for a full set of clubs, but we wanted to give you a little bit of science to think about when it comes to choosing your own clubs. Tour players don't buy their equipment "off the rack," so don't underestimate the power of a proper Tour-style golf club fitting. Hopefully, it'll be in the back of your mind that as your body becomes more optimized for the game, you might want to think about that vital last link in the chain of events that make up the golf swing.

To get the most out of your body on the course, it's also important to think about what you're putting into your body on the course. You want to hydrate and fuel yourself properly while you play. This isn't a nutrition book. We're not going to break down your individual protein, carbohydrate, and fat needs and then micromanage what your sources for each should be. What we are going to do is give you some tips for keeping your body running optimally while you play.

And we're going to start with hydration. You need to stay hydrated on the course. You can probably survive five hours without eating while you play – although you won't be playing your best – but you just cannot go without hydration for five hours on the course. To put it simply, not eating while you play is foolish, but not hydrating while you play is dangerous.

Your body needs water. It needs it to function properly both physically and mentally. In a dehydrated state, you'll find yourself lacking power, endurance, and possibly experiencing muscle cramps. You'll also be sabotaging your nervous system if you're not drinking enough. Just about everything in this book has been about improving neuromuscular function, so the last thing you want to do is compromise it.

A good rule of thumb is to drink four to six bottles of water over the course of your round. This is going to depend on your size – a smaller person might only need four, while a larger person may need six. It'll also depend on the climate. Here, in Florida, the weather can be brutally hot and humid, so you may need more. An early spring 18 holes in upstate New York may not require as much hydration. The key is to stay ahead of your thirst. If you're thirsty, you're already dehydrated!

Based on the playing conditions and how long you're going to be out in the sun, you might also want to think about water or a sports drink with added electrolytes and minerals. If you go the sports drink route, look for one that doesn't have any added sugars or artificial sweeteners. If you go with straight water, do the environment a favor and bring a reusable bottle that can be refilled throughout the round.

> *"Since working out with Kolby, I feel like the length of my career is going to be a lot longer than it would have been with what I was doing before."*
> – Jaye Marie Green

As far as food goes, you want to stay away from heavy, fatty foods – like a good chunk of the stuff you'll find at the end of the front nine. Interestingly, many of the best golfers on the planet fuel themselves on the course with pretty much the same things you carried in your lunch box as a kid: peanut butter sandwiches and bananas. Both are filling and satisfying without being overly heavy. And as long as you don't crush them under sleeves of balls, both should hold up well over your round as neither requires refrigeration. The sugars in the banana will be tempered by the slower-burning carbohydrates in the sandwich's whole grain bread. The fat in the peanut butter will also help slow sugars from being released too quickly into the bloodstream. This will give you the sustained energy you need over the course of 18 holes. Digging a little deeper into the chemistry of things, the sodium in the peanut butter and bread and the potassium in the banana – combined with all the hydrating that you're doing – will help stave off muscle cramps. And after working so hard to fine-tune and rebalance the musculature of your body, the last thing you want to deal with is a calf or hamstring cramp.

If peanut butter isn't your thing, you can always substitute almond butter or cashew butter. Beware, though. All nut butters are not created equally. Look for brands that have as few ingredients as possible. Ideally, your peanut, almond, or cashew butter shouldn't be made up of much more than peanuts, almonds, or cashews. Stay away from brands that add extra oils or sugars.

If you can't eat nuts, go with the simplest energy bar you can find. The fewer the ingredients, the better. And if you can pronounce all the ingredients, even better! Be careful of bars with chocolate in them. Not only will it have potentially negative effects on your blood sugar levels, it will also be a colossal mess to try to eat on the 15th hole of an 87-degree August day.

> *"I won the U.S. Open in 2009, but today, at 40, I'm swinging the club faster than I ever have and playing better and more consistently than I ever have."*
> – **Lucas Glover**

Thank you for trusting us with your body and your golf game. We know about the power of movement and the power of exercise. We both have built and rebuilt our own bodies with reasoned, science-based philosophies and protocols. And we both spend our days helping others optimize their bodies based on these same principles and applications. All we have to do is look up at all the banners we've hung to know that what we do works.

All we ask from you is your effort, your hard work, and your dedication. Get ready to trust the process. Get ready to enjoy the grind. Get ready to play the best golf of your life. Trust, train, and win.

Nothing is impossible when you're armed with a proven plan and the tools, the determination, and the drive to see that plan all the way to fruition.

If you were standing in the Joey D Golf Sports Training Center right now, you'd see the best golfers in the world going through the same exercises and drills that are now part of your golf life. They do them because their careers depend on playing golf at the highest level possible. They do them because they all dream of being number one in the world – and three of them have made that dream a reality. And there's no reason why you can't follow their lead and start to play the game at a level you've only dreamed of.

All right. We've talked long enough. Now go out and hang some banners of your own.

Ready for More?

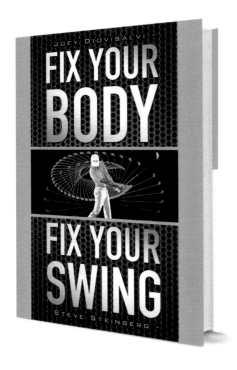

FIX YOUR BODY, FIX YOUR SWING

amazon.com

Coach Joey D's first book is a trouble-shooting guide for the golfer's body.

Readers learn physical assessments that determine where a golfer's body is too tight, not strong enough, or out of balance. Then discover specific, easy-to-follow exercises that correct whatever problems or limitations were revealed in the assessments.

Just three 20-minute workout sessions a week (only one hour a week!) will help anyone become a better golfer with a healthier, stronger body.

HIT IT GREAT®
Online Training Programs
hititgreat.com

Discover great golf fitness training programs from Coach Joey D, Coach Kolby Tullier, and other phenomenal experts streaming online and through apps for iOS and Android.

Designed for players at all levels working at home or in the gym, choose from a growing library of dynamic, easy-to-follow videos and gain more flexibility, speed, power, and distance!

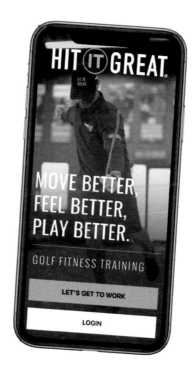

Acknowledgments

I've met and had the support of many amazing, talented, and wonderful people on this journey – far too many to include in this small space. I appreciate each and every one of you for the support, opportunity, education, and friendship.

For the players I've been fortunate to befriend and train, thank you. You are the reason this book exists and why our profession is validated. I'm proud of every one of you.

Thank you, Butch Harmon. You've been a great mentor to me. I'm a much better coach for knowing you.

Thanks to Stephanie and Mark for helping build the platform our team can stand on to help golfers feel and play better. You guys are amazing.

To my daughter, Harper. Thank you for your endless love and patience. You are my greatest gift and my whole heart.

Thank you, Carley. You are my forever love. Thank you for believing in me and us. And Madison and Olivia for trusting me in your lives.
–Joey Diovisalvi, October 2020

This book is dedicated to my parents, Brad and Karen. Thank you for always believing in me and believing that I could accomplish anything with hard work and dedication. All I ever wanted was to make you proud of me.

To my wife, Tracy, my rock. Thank you for allowing me to chase this dream and showing me what love and support truly mean and for being on the journey with me.

To my daughter, Kamryn, for giving me the best blessing in my life, being your dad. I hope you never stop dreaming and chasing the stars.

To each and every one of my clients. Thank you for allowing me to work with you and be a part of your fitness journey. I would not be here without you. This book is for you.
–Kolby Tullier, October 2020

Thanks to Joey and Kolby for their continued friendship and their trust in letting me help get their message out. Thanks to all their players for being so open and willing to talk. Thanks to Mark and everyone else at the Joey D Golf Sports Training Center for being so helpful. And thanks to these folks: Farnold, Jie, Michele, Rujing, Tania, and Tim.
–Steve Steinberg, October 2020

About the Authors

Joey Diovisalvi has been elevating the games of pro athletes for over 30 years and has been working with PGA and LPGA golfers for over 20 years. He's the first strength, conditioning, and biomechanics coach in PGA Tour history to help three players reach number one in the Official World Golf Rankings.

Kolby Tullier has been working with elite athletes for over 20 years. His athletes have won Player of the Year awards on both the PGA Tour and LPGA Tour and reached number one in the Official World Golf Rankings, won the World Series and played in MLB's All-Star game, and won the Super Bowl and played in the NFL's Pro Bowl.

Steve Steinberg has been in the fitness industry as a teacher, trainer, and writer for over 20 years. He's the owner of Charles River Fitness in Waltham, Massachusetts. *Hang the Banner* is his third book.